3.22.2022

COVID BYTES

NAKED MUSINGS OF A DISEASE DETECTIVE

All best wishes!

LAMAR HASBROUCK, MD, MPH, MBA
FOREWORD BY ROBERT E. FULLILOVE, EdD

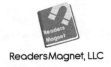

ReadersMagnet, LLC

CONTENTS

The COVID-19 pandemic has been long, difficult, and impactful, in so many ways, to so many different people. Few observations of this once-in-a-lifetime event are as thoughtful as those of Dr. LaMar Hasbrouck's in COVID BYTES: Naked Musings of a Disease Detective. With lived experience, and a life devoted to addressing disparities and fighting diseases, Dr. Hasbrouck moves from standard "doctor talk" to an almost day-by-day mix of key information and humorous but real observations about COVID that make this both a quick page-turner that we can all identify with, laugh and cry about, and see ourselves in...as well as a meaningful and critical historic piece that we can all learn from.

--Joseph Betancourt, MD, MPH, Senior Vice President, Equity and Community Health, Massachusetts General Hospital

COVID BYTES is a fascinating blow-by-blow account of the most serious pandemic in modern history. As seen through the eyes of an experienced disease hunter it chronicles the pandemic in a way that no one else has. There are many books on this global tragedy but none capture the pandemic in real time as Dr. Hasbrouck has. It is an informative read for anyone interested in the evolution of this pandemic and the U.S. response over time.

--Georges C. Benjamin, MD, Executive Director, American Public Health Association

This poignant chronicle of our nation's journey in COVID embodies the phrase "reach out and touch somebody's hand - - make this world a better place if you can." This book reaches out and touches us in so many important ways. It provides accessible truths without evoking fear. It presents a strident hologram of COVID, allowing us to see it from many different angles over time. And, the bedside manner Dr. Hasbrouck employs in delivering narratives of the many shades of COVID calms our spirit to the point of reflection with purpose to transcend a dark time in human-kind. This book is a must read for everyone who wants to understand the COVID experience in real time and how it has shaped our world and our everyday lives. It is, in fact, an exceptional read from a highly knowledgeable health advocate who walks in truth and social justice.

--Dr. Linda M. Burton, Dean, School of Social Welfare, University of California, Berkeley

The straightforward and informed advice that chronicles the unfolding of the COVID-19 pandemic is both compelling and engaging. The scorching candor provides a noted expert's critical review of the political and social issues that continue to impede the public's health in America. "COVID Bytes" provides case-study gold for public health educators seeking to train the next generation of leaders in our field.

--Crystal M. James, JD, MPH, Special Assistant to the President for COVID-19 Recovery, Co-Director Center for Rural Health & Economic Equity, Head, Dept. Graduate Public Health, Tuskegee University

What a delightful read chronicling the pandemic. This is such an easy read. I am impressed with your (Dr. Hasbrouck's) formatting of the pandemic. Your (His) blow-by-blow chronicle of the pandemic provides the reader with the feeling that they are right there with you (him). This work will provide information and perspective for the lay public to better understand where we were in the epidemic.

--*Dr. C. Perry Brown, Professor of Public Health, Florida A&M University*

DEDICATION

This book is dedicated to the more than 600,000 Americans who perished from COVID-19.

For epidemiologists and "disease detectives" everywhere who protect the health and safeguard the lives of people in all corners of the world.

And, to the health care workers, first responders, and essential workers that enabled us to keep our heads above water, even at great risk to themselves and their families.

"What matters most is how well you walk through the fire."

— Charles Bukowski

FOREWORD

I first met LaMar Hasbrouck in 1986. He was about to enter the Master of Public Health degree program at the University of California, Berkeley, but his eyes were on a much more important credential. He was clear that the master's degree was going to be the stepping stone to a career that would blend the science of public health with the healing arts of clinical medicine. He completed the MPH, made his way to medical training at UCLA, followed that with residencies in New York at NY Presbyterian Cornell Weil, and became an Epidemic Intelligence Service Officer at the Centers for Disease Control and Prevention. He traveled extensively and worked many of the "hotspots" internationally, engaged in battling Ebola and a host of other viral threats to the human family.

Those would have served as an impressive foundation for a faculty position in a medical school setting, but he was not done. He has held leadership positions that included becoming the 17th Director of the Illinois Department of Public Health and the Chief Executive Officer at the National Association of County and City

Health Officials. Having grown up in what might be described as "modest circumstances," his rise to become a leader of US medicine and public health provides him with a unique focus to understand the worldwide devastation of COVID-19.

Early on in his career, I had numerous opportunities to observe him in action. The more I watched, the more I became convinced that I was observing a Black doctor from the Old School. Here was a 21st-century physician engaged in patient-doctor interactions that sang loudly and clearly of another era, when doctors were defined by their bedside manner, not their medical school admissions scores or their published works. Medical science has evolved far beyond the point of being understandable or accessible to members of the general public. In many clinical practice settings, it is not the physician who communicates with patients but rather a health educator or a physician's assistant. In such places, talking to the patient is a lost art, a fond memory of the good old days.

What a wondrous surprise awaits the reader of COVID BYTES. My star MPH candidate and medical school scholar has evolved. Moreover, he has written a chronicle of the COVID-19 pandemic where he fills a much-needed void. He manages to breakdown the complexity of the pandemic and in his best, old-fashioned Black doctor's voice, he makes clear what was much too often left cloudy by inept and often inaccurate reporting from the Centers for Disease Control. Those of us who know and work with the CDC knew only too well that the voice of science was being actively and criminally silenced by the White House. We sympathized with their dilemma and their inability to overcome a president whose fondness for half-truths and rumors was placing all of us at risk.

It was left to Dr. LaMar to explain what our public officials were unable to articulate. Reading his event-to-event chronicling of the pandemic in this book is a wonderful exercise in taking the complexities of the pandemic and rendering them accessible. His writing comes at a time when public health researchers and officials have made tremendous strides in understanding the dynamics of COVID-19 and its impact on the individual's body as well on the bodies of an entire nation. However, what he makes clear is that the ability to discuss and explain that knowledge to the public is sorely lacking.

In too many instances throughout the worst days of the pandemic, public health officials would release a report on some key aspects of our struggles to stay ahead of COVID-19. We would learn, for instance, that fully vaccinated persons did not need to wear a mask for most indoor and outdoor gatherings. The statement was based on countless hours of analyzing data about the risk of transmission of the virus as well as the risks of contracting it. But when the announcement was made with great fanfare, the person in the street had no idea what action was supposed to be taken based on that finding. "Can we stop wearing masks?" "Does that mean that if I am vaccinated and some creep insists I put on my mask, I can yell back 'I'm vaccinated,' and they will leave me alone?"

COVID BYTES is a book that works very hard to avoid those miscommunications. With elegant ease and patience, Dr. LaMar's blogs throughout the year 2020 would pick up all of the sources of confusion embedded in these 'official pronouncements.' His entries would slowly but surely explain step by step what it all means, why it is being announced, or, better, what the pronouncement did NOT mean. In anticipating the level of fear that would be raised by a cryptic official communication, he spent the year putting it all into perspective. In the manner of the old fashion doc with a polished bedside manner, he not only made it clear, but he also voiced calmly when calm was called for. And when trouble was looming in the midst of the statistics and trend data, he made clear why he would be exercising great caution in unpacking the science of epidemiological predictions.

His understanding of the need for skillful communicators is particularly present when he writes, "Crisis communication is key during times of, well, crisis. During stressful times people want an honest broker of the facts. You can never communicate too much, AND consistency, accuracy, and timeliness are all paramount."

Reading COVID BYTES is to be in the presence of such an honest broker of the facts. Our lives have been irrevocably changed by this pandemic. In this week-to-week chronicle of our struggles with COVID, we see clearly how the crisis evolved. We see through his writing the missteps, the misunderstandings of the nature of the challenge we were facing, but there is also the gradual, steady progress towards a vaccine and eventually, a way out.

We all lived through it. As you read COVID BYTES, you will now have a unique opportunity to put it all in perspective. In the process of making sense of what we've endured, Dr. LaMar has also given us the tools to learn from our traumas and unite in the so vitally necessary work of healing the horrors that befell us all.

Robert E. Fullilove, EdD
Professor and Associate Dean
Columbia University Mailman School of Public Health

ACKNOWLEDGMENTS

To my parents Jim and Beverly Tolbert who poured into me and provided me with a solid foundation from which to launch my creative endeavors, personal development pursuits, and passion projects. Thank you for your resolute support and listening ears. Also, thank you for getting vaccinated.

To my daughters (and legacy) Baele Simone, Maysa Farai, and Lalah Rose who inspire me to maximize my manhood as a father every day. You girls give my life special meaning and value and joy. It has been a gift to witness each of you step into young womanhood with courage, character, conviction, and compassion while doggedly pursuing your dreams.

To Hagir Elawad, my partner in service, for your encouragement, advice, copy editing, out loud performance readings, unsolicited candid advice, and good humor. I am convinced that you are the second funniest person on our team.

To my siblings, immediate family, and family Zoomers, including Jaeneen Johnson, LaSalle Hasbrouck, Marvin A. Smith, Jem Turman, Carita Turman, Natalie Johnson,

James Johnson, Nicole Jones, Delano Jones, Victoria Jones, Christian Jones, Alexandya Fountain, Karrengton Fountain, Jay Turman, Susan Turman, Rage' Richardson, Kathy Sanders, Karen Gill, Deborah Garbey, Mitchell Howard, Nell Anderson, Brenda Webster, Lauren Webster, and others. Historically, our visits were limited to my infrequent visits to my hometown of San Diego, CA. One small silver lining of the pandemic was that it brought us together for monthly check-ins. Our hearty discussions about all things COVID, politics related to health access, and social justice, kept me grounded in the realities of everyday people and pushed me to provide the best information possible. We are a resilient tribe indeed.

To my mentors past and present on whose shoulders I stand. They have challenged me to explore my intellectual curiosity while being of service to the community. To Bob E. Fullilove, Reed V. Tuckson, Perry Brown, David Satcher, Bill Jenkins, John Rich, Mindy Fullilove, Holly Andersen, and others, thank you for setting such a high standard of excellence and having my back. And to my early educators at the UC Berkeley School of Public Health (Patricia Morgan, Lee Riley, Raul Caetano, Art Reingold, Denise Herd, and Cathy Kodama) and the Centers for Disease Control and Prevention (Douglas Hamilton, Alex Crosby, Steven Thacker, Bill Murrain, Tim Thornton, and James Mercy).

I am grateful to the media mavens from large and small markets, including journalists, producers, and editors that magnified my voice, allowing me to contribute to the national conversation in a substantive way. Specifically, I want to recognize Jayne O'Donnell, Cydney Henderson, Carly Mallenbaum with USA Today; Brianna Keilar, Kate Bolduan, Ted Metzger, Steven Page, and Marie Malzberg with CNN; Joe Mahr with Chicago Tribune; Josh Kovensky and Kate Riga with Talking Points Memo; Gerren Keith Gaynor with TheGrio; Selena Simmons-Duffin with NPR; Leslie Goldman with Vox; Alex Vuocolo with Cheddar News; Ali Pattillo with Inverse; Juandolyn Stokes with News-Talk 1380; Hannah Kliger with News12, Bronx; James Bikales with CalMatters; Jeff D'Alessio with The News-Gazette; and, Candace Y.A. Montague with the Center for Health Journalism. Also, thanks to publications that carried my opinions during the past year, including The Hill, San Francisco Chronicle, The Business Journal, and numerous others.

I must acknowledge the most avid followers of my LinkedIn series called CoronaWatch: Doc Talk with Dr. LaMar. Without your persistent curiosity and active and thoughtful engagement my posting may have been sporadic at best. Thank you to Adaeze Okorafor, Andrew Christler, Anne-Marie Burton, Antoinette Bragg, Antoniah Lewis-Reese, Bahby Banks, Barkley Payne, Brenda Jones, Brian McGhee, Camilla Johnson, Celeste R. Davis. Chantel Wilcox, Charlene Wells, Chester Charles, II, Claire Rosche Matzzie, Connie Boatman-Tate, Crystal Swann, Damon Green, Danielle Lazar, Darryl Stallworth, David Elin, David Leit, David Miller, David Ortega, Deneen Sarlas, Dennis Small, Diana P. Linero, Diane Clay, Edrewnae Lewis, Einas Ahmed, Elliott Auerbach, Erica Cunningham, Francisco Nunez, Gabriela Illa, George W.

Roberts, Gita Rampersad, Harold Jolley, Hope King, James Devers, Jamie Burns, Jamyia Clark, Janel Hughes-Jones, Jill M. Humphries, JoBeth McCarthy, Joe Smyser, Josephine Ansah, Justin DeJong, Kate Vergara, Katrina Rhodes, Kecia Washington, Kenneth J. Jones, II, Kevin Reddy, Larry Hancock, LaShannon Spencer, Laura M. Jacobs, Leslie Bender, Lisa Aponte-Soto, Lorri Jenkins, Lubna Jamal, Marcus A. Williams, Margaret Mueller, Maria Jones, Marilyn Green, Mark Hunter, Marvin Bembry, Mathilda Lambert, Megan Davis, Melissa Funderburk, Melissa Hagan, Michael Jones, Michael Mendoza, Michael Orquiza, Michael Penn, Montrece Ransom, Nadeen Chambers, NaNotchka Chumley, Nasseam James, Nat'e Russell, Nicola Williams, Nicole F. Roberts, Nicole L. Curtis, Nycal Anthony-Townsend, Oscar Alleyne, Peter R. Hubbard, Philip M. J. Baptist, Rachel Sacks, Ray Wang, Rebecca Krueger, Rodrigo A. Sierra, Rosalyn Casas, Rosie D. Lyles, Sabrina Nelson, Samuel Jarvis, Sara Berg, Schara Dassie, Sean Murphy, Serene Bridgett Hollingsworth, Shane Scott, Siji Varghese, Sinan Almukhtar, Sonja Rasmussen, Sophie Michals, Stephanie Hasan, Tanya Lopez, Tatia Hodges, Theresa Wukusick, Tia Christian-Hunt, Tricia Mosley, Uzoamaka Nwafor, Wendell Peoples, and many others, among the thousands who followed in stealth mode.

I also want to recognize and salute my colleagues who freely contributed to educating the public about the pandemic. It was hard at times to penetrate the white noise of the pandemic chatter given the avalanche of opinions however well informed. Individual health heroes who embraced the challenge of counterbalancing misinformation with both evidence-based practice and practice-based evidence, include Camara Jones, Bechara Choucair, Denise Fair, Esther Choo, Jay Bhatt, John Whyte, Joneigh S. Khaldun, Julie Morita, Leana Wen, Lisa K. Fitzpatrick, Marcell Nunez-Smith, Oni Blackstock, Rick Bright, and Uche' Blackstock. Organizations and campaigns that were out front include the Chicago Urban League, BlackDoctor. org, Black Coalition Against COVID, the Greater Than COVID campaign, and Grapevine Health.

To the scores of mentees that I have connected with over the past three decades, including those that have recently entrusted me to be a mentor, Amy Ekhaguere, Karsyn Terry, Kortni Washington, Tyler Jackson, Zinn Amos, I encourage you to find and use your voice to make a difference as you prepare to take the baton as health leaders in the future.

I can't leave out the late-night show hosts like Seth Meyers, Stephen Colbert, Samantha Bee, and Trevor Noah. Their sobering satirical insights inspired me to take a closer look at the ripple effects of pandemic. I am convinced that a spoon full of comedy helps the medicine go down.

Finally, I want to recognize Maria Loradel Madeja and the rest of the publication team from ReadersMagnet for helping me to assemble this book for distribution to the interested masses.

Book jacket design by Derry Frima.
Author photo by Shaun Michael at Year 2139.

PREFACE

How did we get here? It's hard to remember the old normal. We long for a simpler time when you could greet a person with a handshake or a hug. You could dine in a restaurant or see a movie in the theater without a second thought. Kids and parents discussed taking the bus, the car, or walking to school, not whether they would go back in person. It was a time when work meetings were conducted in a conference room not so much by conference call, and teams were what you called small groups working together, not a video-conference program by the same name.

The novel coronavirus turned the world upside down. This new virus proved to be a formidable threat for an unsuspecting nation led to denial by a president incapable of meeting the moment. As the pandemic swept across America, we lost precious time that we would never get back. From December 2019 through March 2020, we sat on our hands. Eventually, the country transitioned from a defensive posture of travel bans and cruise ship concerns to mitigating guidance, albeit inconsistent. Finally, in the early part of 2021, our national response progressed to a successful vaccination campaign under a new administration.

As many Americans were left scratching their heads in response to the foreign lexicon of epidemics, it became apparent that a translator would be helpful. I decided to gingerly step into this void on LinkedIn. I kept it simple. And by the second week, I had a devoted following hungry to better understand the shifting landscape, and eager to read my insights. With the rapidly evolving situation and repeated cringe-worthy gaffes by the leadership, I kept on sharing. A year later, I had posted on more than 150 days, sometimes multiple times a day.

I opined about testing, differential impact on racial minorities, herd immunity, financial bailouts, celebrity transmissions, questionable therapies, and superspreading events to name a few. Each post was packed into the 1,300-character limit (200 words) allotted. Thus, every post was a byte-sized, easily consumable, informational nugget. This book compiles the 100 posts with the most reactions. Hopefully, reading them will cause you to ponder. You may even chuckle on occasion. But more than anything, I hope these COVID bytes spur dialogue that will nudge our collective education to a place that better equips us for the next pandemic.

When the dust settles, coronavirus will be remembered as one of the greatest public health threats in our nation's history. It will be remembered as a season of missed opportunities, unprecedented fear, and collective anxiety. In our new normal, we relate to one another across the buffer of social distance and through the barrier of face masks. Inconvenienced and fatigued, we go about our daily routines with cautious consideration. For many, the new normal is one of practical self-preservation. For others, it is one of entitled defiance to preserve individual liberties.

At the time of this writing, our world remains in the grip of the COVID-19. By summoning our humanity, we can cross this chasm of profound loss. The incalculable loss of jobs, income, freedoms, peace of mind, and void of loved ones that perished. It sounds corny, I know, but we are all in this together. We are a melting pot of the fringed vulnerable and the worried well. A gumbo of the empowered and skeptical. Our fates are interlaced and in order to defeat this scourge, we will need to harness the best of who we are.

INTRODUCTION

Everyone enjoys watching their favorite sports competition on TV. But we rarely, if ever, watch with the volume muted. If we did, chances are we would not enjoy it as much. We would miss the grunts Serena makes when she hits her backhand returns and the roar of the crowd after a Steph Curry 3-pointer. But we'd also miss something else: the commentary from the expert analyst. Both the play-by-play announcer and the quick-witted color commentator add to our experience. The former describes what we're seeing. The latter helps us better understand what we're seeing by putting it into context with humor, sarcasm, and forecasting outcomes. Because of their insider's knowledge and their relatable communication style, the value-added from these sage guides is welcomed by even the most ardent fans. But if you're a newbie unfamiliar with the sport, they are as valuable as a flashlight during a power outage at night. Without them, we would be utterly lost.

COVID-19 seemed to come out of nowhere. Of course, it had been smoldering in China for months before it arrived in the states. This type of virus was not new to infectious disease experts, epidemiologists, and researchers. However, for the vast majority of the public, it was foreign in every way. The tsunami of information, challenges, and life-changing mandates were inconceivable. Prior to COVID, the term quarantine was most often used to refer to pets undergoing precautions for rabies. Terms like isolation, contact tracing, flattening the curve, and herd immunity were all Greek to most.

What is contained herein are the real-time opinions (or "naked musings") of an expert with behind-the-scenes knowledge and actual experience in both planning for and responding to disease outbreaks. During the first year (and 500,000 deaths) of the COVID pandemic, I acted as both play-by-play analyst and color commentator for a lay audience experiencing unchartered waters. I did so, not as a source of entertainment, but in an effort to inform and guide an inexperienced public through the storm. The content is not based on my contemporaneous notes weaved together after the fact. Rather, it is a compilation of 100 of my actual posts that reached tens of thousands of people through LinkedIn, the professional networking platform.

My process was uncomplicated and unfiltered. I tracked our nation's response by reading and listening to the daily reporting, changing government guidelines, and reflecting on the wisdom, missed opportunities, or blunders. Simply stated, I learned, reflected, and then posted. What resulted was a string of concise analyses about the actions, reactions, or non-actions. My commentary covered a range of topics from convalescent antibodies to celebrity infections, coping with social isolation, even rogue politicians.

Few of us were around for the Spanish flu in 1918 that killed nearly 700,000. But most of us can recall the H1N1 pandemic of 2009 that took the lives of about 12,000 Americans. At the time, I was running a county health department in upstate New York. So, I have been through the pandemic drill before, albeit on a smaller scale. Managing that threat required studying table-top mock scenarios, forecasting hospital bed capacity, and conducting live mass casualty drills with first responders. We mobilized volunteer health professionals, and vaccinated thousands of residents in school gymnasiums and at pop-up clinics. Luckily, we met the moment.

I have had many opportunities to respond to outbreaks. Much of this experience was gained working at the Centers for Disease Control and Prevention (CDC). My induction into the CDC began as a fellow in the Epidemic Intelligence Service (EIS). As an EIS Officer or disease detective, I learned from some of the smartest scientists in the world. I put this knowledge to the test when dispatched around the globe to track down infectious outbreaks and other emerging public health threats. During my 11-year tenure there, I tackled West Nile Virus, smallpox, monkeypox, polio, and HIV. Assignments sent me to Haiti, Bangladesh, Nigeria, Namibia, Vietnam, and many other destinations prior to directing the CDC office in Guyana, South America.

Some years later, I had the opportunity to run the health department for the State of Illinois. As fate would have it, protecting the health and safety of 13 million residents included managing responses to novel influenza outbreaks, vaccine shortages, the Middle East Respiratory Syndrome (MERS), and quarterbacking the game plan against the deadly Ebola virus as the Governor-appointed co-chair of the statewide Ebola Task Force.

These experiences proved one thing. And that is, the approach to an infectious disease outbreak is fundamentally the same irrespective of the scenario. Every response requires risk assessment, testing, mitigation strategies, ongoing monitoring (i.e., surveillance), public education, and crisis communication. In other words, there is a playbook. I have used it many times. I guess the gravity of the moment compelled me to share my thoughts with the world. Reading them won't make you an epidemiologist, but it will give you insights into how one thinks.

I made every effort to be balanced and objective. Admittedly, the occasional post may have been colored by my profound disappointment with the guidance offered by a few members of the White House Coronavirus Task Force, some of whom I have worked with professionally and known for years. That said, my goal was neither to offer definitive solutions nor to second-guess the policy positions by the officials put in charge. Rather, my purpose was to provoke options that could result in better policy-making and more accountable personal decisions.

As a country, we lost big. Notwithstanding the damage to our collective psyche, shattered social lives, or strained pocketbooks, we lost 600,000-plus lives.

For these reasons, we cannot afford to lose the lessons. Beyond its entertainment value, COVID BYTES is worth reading because it simultaneously chronicles our nation's response (e.g., guidance, experimental therapies, Project Warp Speed) to the worst pandemic in a hundred years. It also gives historical voice to the myriad of unintended consequences of the response.

The content in the book is organized into five sections. There is a short preamble followed by four parts that correspond to the seasonal shifts in the pandemic. Every 200-word post ends with a statistical line that shows the number of COVID cases (both global and US), deaths (global and the US), and the overall death rate (or case fatality rate), abbreviated CFR. The stat line summarizes the severity of the pandemic on the day of my posting. My source for the estimates was The New York Times interactive coronavirus world map.

Finally, a word about the intended audience. Obviously, every author wants their book to be read by the broadest audience possible. I am no different. But in addition to the general audience, I predict a keen interest by students in public health, population health, nursing, and other allied health professions. Moreover, I see great value for graduate students in epidemiology, medicine, global health, healthcare management, policy, and administration. COVID has laid bare the fact that the real-world application of scientific knowledge is swayed by politics, economic constraints, and public trust. This important lesson, though devoid from most curriculum, is worth learning.

In any case, I hope that you enjoy the book and I want to hear from you. Please visit my website at www. drlamarmd.org or message me on LinkedIn. I welcome your feedback and look forward to interacting with you, even if it means being respectfully challenged.

PREAMBLE: WINTER WORRY

On January 9, the World Health Organization (WHO) announced a mysterious coronavirus illness-causing pneumonia in Wuhan, China. With the threat seemingly a world away, Americans were unphased and unconcerned. Less than two weeks later, the CDC confirmed the first US case of coronavirus, a traveler from Wuhan. It was a resident in Washington state. CDC dispatches a team of disease detectives to investigate. Before the month would end, WHO would issue a global health emergency after exponential growth in cases around the globe. Unable to ignore the growing death toll of more than 200, a few days later, on February 3, the Trump administration declared a nationwide public health emergency. Despite his reassuring tone, worry begins to mount as the global case count approaches 10,000.

This novel coronavirus was not declared a pandemic at that point, but it was clearly heading in that direction. A slew of questions from family members, colleagues, and friends prompted me to launch an informational blog on February 26. I called it CoronaWatch: Doc Talk with Dr. LaMar. My eyes were peeled wide open for sure. However, the engagement with others on LinkedIn fueled me to exercise my mental muscles as a former CDC Disease Detective. I begin the series with basic terms and information about influenza-like illnesses.

Series Introduction

Feb. 26, 2020

In today's small world, an outbreak anywhere is a potential outbreak everywhere! I've been on the front line in response to West Nile, novel flu (e.g., H1N1), SARS, MERS, Ebola, and Zika. Today's outbreak du jour: novel coronavirus. In this series of posts, I'll tell you what you need to know in easy-to-understand language and provide updates as the pandemic unfolds.

Post #1: Flu Basics

Feb. 27, 2020

First, a few basics. Every year about 10% of the US population (36 million) get the seasonal flu and up to 60,000 dies as a result. However, unlike the seasonal flu that peaks from Dec. – Feb. for which we have an annual vaccine, coronavirus has no seasonal pattern and there is no vaccine. Unfortunately, it will take more than a year to develop a vaccine for this bug. And that's vaccine development on the fast track! Coronavirus is a new (or novel) virus that hasn't been previously seen in humans. That's why there's no vaccine. COVID-19, which stands for COrona-VIrus-Disease-2019, is related to other viruses that have caused outbreaks in recent years (SARS, MERS). The infection causes mild to severe flu-like symptoms (fever, cough, shortness of breath) and can be deadly. The virus spreads easily by breathing in virus-laden droplets (mist from coughing, sneezing, even talking), and can probably be picked up from contaminated surfaces. It takes 2 days to 2 weeks for people to show symptoms. This time lag is called the incubation period.

Case count: 82,130 (US, 60); Deaths: 2,796 (US, 0); CFR: 3.4%

Post #2: Is the Threat Real or Imagined?

Feb. 28, 2020

The threat is real, but lowish, for now. Risk is determined by several factors: 1) circulation of the virus in a community; 2) ease of spread; 3) disease severity, and 4) vulnerability of the person infected. Currently, the virus is not widely spread in the US, but we had the first community-acquired case. This is alarming because previously all infections were "imported" by travelers from "hot zones". COVID-19, like seasonal flu, appears highly contagious. Stand w/n 3-feet of an infected person that sneezes and there's a good chance you'll get it. Severity is measured by the case fatality rate (CFR). Simply put, this is the proportion of people who die from a specified disease. The CFR for COVID-19 is ~3% (Math check: 2,858 deaths/83,655 cases x 100 = 3.4%). Compare this w/ seasonal flu (0.1%), SARS (15%), MERS (34%). While it's 30x more deadly than the flu, it's nowhere near as deadly as these other infections. Lastly, one's immune system is important. Those with weakened immune systems are at the highest risk. For example, people 70+ years or w/ heart disease have a much higher death rate (~10%) vs. those younger than 49 years or without preexisting conditions (~1%).

Case Count: 83,655 (US, 60); Deaths: 2,858 (US, 0); CFR: 3.4%

Post #3: Personal Protection

Feb. 29, 2020

The adage "an ounce of prevention is worth a pound of cure" holds true. Despite a vaccine being at least a year away, it's never too early for an "education inoculation." Practice the 3 C's: Clean, Cover, and Contain. Wash your hands often or use alcohol-based hand sanitizer. Cover your cough and sneeze with a tissue, then discard it. Contain the illness by avoiding close contact w/ people who are sick or isolating yourself if you're sick. Remember, people are most contagious when they have symptoms. Masks should be worn by people who are sick to prevent further spread, rather than by healthy people trying to avoid infection. This helps preserve the stockpiles of masks for healthcare workers and first responders. Avoiding crowds and mass gatherings may be a good idea. Certainly, when there's more community spread it's wise to reconsider elective activities such as children's play dates, movie outings, even worship services. Lastly, avoid traveling to places where there is widespread community transmission. CDC gives 3 risk levels for travel: Level 1-Be careful; Level 2-Reconsider; Level 3-Avoid.

Case Count: 85,400 (US, 64); Deaths: 2,921 (US, 1); CFR: 3.8%

Total COVID-19 deaths in the U.S. through February 2020

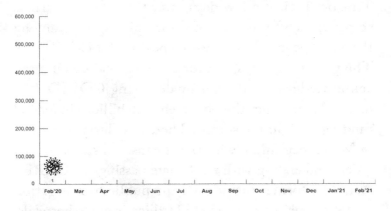

Source: Worldometer

PART 1: SPRING FORWARD

The epidemic continues to ramp up and is officially declared a pandemic by the WHO on March 11. This occurs just a few days after the infamous cruise ship arrives off the coast of California carrying among the 3,500 people dozens testing positive for COVID-19. The threat becomes real for all Americans as Trump acknowledges the danger by declaring COVID-19 a national emergency thereby freeing up billions in federal funding to fight the spread. There is a flurry of actions in March beginning with travel bans and stay-at-home orders and ending with the Senate passing the CARES Act. The former introduced the public to mitigation strategies, the latter provided $2 trillion in aid to hospitals, state and local governments, and small businesses.

The nation was also introduced to the malaria and arthritis drug, hydroxychloroquine, as the president posed the question "What do you have to lose?" by taking the unproven drug. Spring was notable for a precipitous rise in the epi-curve and US deaths hit the 100,000 mark by late May. Despite infections among celebrities and professional athletes, adherence to social distancing and other precautions began to wane, foreshadowing a term that would epitomize our greatest challenge in defeating the pandemic, "COVID fatigue."

During this season, I posted at a frantic snap. The public seemed to have an increased appetite for learning about the virus and how best to protect themselves, perhaps most pressing, when they could anticipate it all being over. In addition to my posts, I was among the recognized experts asked to opine on a range of related topics. I addressed public health funding, rules for social distancing, the intersection of poverty and COVID, vaccine development, the pandemic playbook, the government's response, and how to safely return to the workplace, appearing on CNN and in publications like the USA Today, Chicago Tribune, Vox, and The Hill.

Post #4: Healthy Workplace

Mar. 2, 2020

There's been much talk about the potential for disruption of everyday life due to COVID-19. Because most full-time employees go to the office, concerns about transmission at work are warranted. Viruses spread easily in close quarters like offices. COVID-19 is no different. In addition to practicing the 3 Cs (Cover cough/sneeze, Clean hands, Contain the illness), there are other tips to lower your risk at work. Limit touching your eyes, nose, mouth. This is the primary way to transfer the virus from surfaces. Wipe down your desk and other common areas like telephones, desks, water fountain handles, microwave door handles, and computer keyboards in offices because they contain germs. CDC recommends that employers take proactive steps to reduce transmission by actively encouraging sick workers to stay home; developing non-punitive flexible leave policies (i.e., telecommuting options); separating sick employees who may become sick during the workday; routine cleaning frequently touched surfaces in common areas (i.e., copy/print area); and curtailing employee travel to large meetings and higher risk countries.

Case Count: 89,732 (US, 88); Deaths: 3,056 (US, 2); CFR: 3.4%

Post #5: Federal Response: Too Little, Too Late?

Mar. 3, 2020

For public health emergencies like COVID-19, there is a proactive and a reactive approach. Proactive is always better. We call this preparedness. This entails having a response plan, equipment/supplies, drilling, trained staff, and if possible, a cadre of volunteers to activate for "surge capacity." Of course, sustained readiness requires sustained investment. Despite the proposed knee-jerk $7 billion packages for this emerging pandemic, Congressional funding for the nation's public health infrastructure, and preparedness specifically, has drastically declined over the past decade or more. This result: flat-footed delays or hectic scrambling by local and state health authorities in response to public health threats. Both pose a public health risk. Leaders in the field have urged federal officials to establish an emergency contingency fund for times like this, but without success. In the @USATODAY article below, I join other experts in clarifying the resource challenges faced where the rubber meets the road.

. Case Count: 92,140 (US, 103); Deaths: 3,125 (US, 6); CFR: 3.4%

Post #6: Boosting Immunity

Mar. 4, 2020

Epidemiologists talk about disease transmission in terms of something called the epidemiologic triad: the agent (virus), the host (people), and the environment (in which the virus and people are brought together). I've discussed the bug and minimizing environmental risk (e.g., cleaning surfaces, social distancing). Now let's discuss YOU, the host. Given the absence of a vaccine or medication for COVID-19, a healthy immune system can help protect you and speed recovery from infection. Ways to boost your immunity include adequate sleep, minimizing stress, don't smoke, a diet high and fresh fruits and veggies, vitamin C, and regular exercise. For many, exercise happens at their neighborhood gym, health club, or yoga studio. Given the current outbreak, is it wise to frequent places seemingly teeming with crowds of sweat-drenched members sharing equipment, grunting, and exhaling in closed spaces? I share tips for staying healthy at the gym in the USA TODAY article below.

Case Count: 94,295 (US, 129); Deaths: 3,210 (US, 9); CFR: 3.4%

Post #7: Counting Matters, Managing Expectations

Mar. 5, 2020

The US has too few cases of COVID-19. We should have more. In fact, I'm confident we DO have more. As the global community approaches 100,000 cases, the US has about 160. How can that be? One theory is our government did a near-perfect job locking COVID-19 out of the country through "air-tight" borders. Unfortunately, viruses pay little attention to travel bands. The truth is we were under-counting. By not testing more widely, we simply don't have the confirmed cases. But they're out there. This phenomenon is known as "surveillance bias" and refers to the idea that the more you look, the more you find, often leading to cases diagnosed more frequently in the more closely monitored group. Reportedly, the US has done about 500 tests in total, yielding 160 cases. Based on the deaths in the US, and the known death rate for COVID-19, we should have approximately 324 cases

(Math check: 11 deaths/.034 CFR = 324). Now that the feds are ramping up testing, expect to see more, lots more. Don't be alarmed. The cases were here all along. Call your HCP to request a test if concerned or at risk.

*Case Count: 95,765 (US, 160); Deaths: 3,281 (US, 11); CFR: 3.4%

Post #8: Funding the Response

Mar. 6, 2020

Cases have now surpassed 100,000 globally and nearly 300 in the US across at least 18 states. Thankfully, our government has finally approved the emergency funding needed to combat the virus. This $8.3 billion supplemental package was approved by a bipartisan Congress and signed by Trump today. Money can buy many things, but it can't buy time. So, quickly putting these resources to work will be vital. State, local, tribal and territorial health departments are not the nimblest when mobilizing funds. Funds are typically routed through CDC to health authorities via grants which takes time. That said, $2.2 billion is earmarked for health agencies, some to replenish diverted funds used for their initial response. In addition, there's $3 billion for the development of vaccines and medicines, more than $800 to increase NIH's capacity, $100 million for community health centers, and $500 million to allow physicians to care for Medicare patients in their homes using telehealth services (e.g., digital remote patient monitoring, consultation), an important strategy given the increased risk for complications among older persons.

Case Count: 101,706 (US, 291); Deaths: 3,456 (US, 15); CFR: 3.4%

Post #9: Breaking Bad

Mar. 7, 2020

As cases continue to predictably rise, more people who were exposed to confirmed cases will be identified. A case is a person with a positive test result. They must be isolated from others to avoid spreading the disease. An exposed person, on the other hand, has NOT been tested. But they have been exposed to a confirmed case (or contact of a case). Persons under investigation (PUI) should be quarantined for 14-days (the incubation period) to ensure they don't develop symptoms. A PUI with symptoms must be tested. A PUI without symptoms need not. Quarantine/isolation can be self-imposed or directed under the local health authority. Both rely on the honor system. When cases (or PUI) break bad and fail to isolate themselves, they put their family and community in harm's way. Rather than breaking the chain of transmission, they add more links. Sadly, people with COVID-19 have been caught slipping out of isolation to attend social events, drive Uber, or take public transportation. Some countries impose jail terms for quarantine evaders. With a healthy dose of community vigilance, it won't come to this here.

Case Count: 105,730 (US, 381); Deaths: 3,559 (US, 19); CFR: 3.4%

Post #10: Fuzzy Math

Mar. 9, 2020

Based on the global fatality rate (3.4%), every death represents about 30 cases. Yet, the US reports 22 deaths, 545 cases. The math is off. Using this formula, we should have 660 cases, 115 more cases! IF you trust the numbers, the fatality rate in the US is higher than the global rate (Math check: 22/545 = 4%). But it's not plausible to have higher death rates in the US compared to the rest of the world. Based on his hunch, Trump claims that the fatality rate is "way under 1%." But we'd need 2,200 cases for this to hold true. You see, it's impossible to have both a low case fatality rate AND few cases without using fuzzy math. Why would our government artificially suppress the numbers? In a word: politics. As an epidemiologist, I am more interested in trusting the numbers than "liking the numbers." Today, the public remains in the dark about the number of Americans being tested. South Korea does 10,000 tests per day. Estimates are that we've done a total of 1,900. Containment of COVID-19 must be based on accurate public health data. We'll never get our arms around this epidemic until our leaders commit to this principle.

Case Count: 109,992 (US, 545); Deaths: 3,825 (22); CFR: 3.5%

Post #11: The 80:20 Rule

Mar. 10, 2020

The 80-20 rule is an often-used expression to describe many things from the qualities of a prospective mate to the productivity of team members, co-insurance, even high need, high-cost patients, so-called super-utilizers. Based on what we've learned so far, we can apply this term to COVID-19. When it comes to the illness for those who are infected, 80% have either mild or no symptoms at all. The illness can look like a bad cold or seasonal flu. For these patients, home isolation, over-the-counter remedies, and remote monitoring by a health professional are enough. For the remaining 20% who may develop severe symptoms (i.e., difficulty breathing) and complications (i.e., pneumonia), these are defined as severe (e.g., requiring oxygen) or critical (e.g., respiratory failure, septic shock). These people may require hospitalization for supportive or intensive care. We can predict who will fall into 20% group. Those at the highest risk are seniors and those with chronic health conditions. Death rates by the numbers are age 80s (15%), 70s (8%), 60s (3.6%); heart disease (11%), diabetes (7%), lung disease, high blood pressure, or cancer (6%).

Case Count: 116,391 (US, 755); Deaths: 4,083 (26); CFR: 3.5%

Post #12: VEEP Gets It, Finally

Mar. 11, 2020

Crisis communication is key during times of, well, crisis. During stressful times people want an honest broker of the facts. You can never communicate too much, and consistency, accuracy, and timeliness are paramount. The spokesperson(s) must be reputable and credible. Admittedly, vice-president Pence's reputation was questionable given his claims that "smoking doesn't kill" and his controversial handling of the worst HIV outbreak in Indiana. But he seems to have learned from those mistakes. Unlike Trump, Pence has consistently put the experts upfront. In a recent press briefing flanked by members of his Coronavirus Task Force, he stated, "there will be more cases." That was the statement I was waiting to hear. He then masterfully directed each technical question from the press to the most appropriate subject matter expert. "He finally gets it," I thought. As a result, I witnessed a lighter, less pensive, posture from the press corps. Even a few moments of collective levity. There's something almost medicinal about honesty. A pandemic is no time for deception. Indeed, "sunlight is the best antiseptic."

Case Count: 121,697 (US, 1,015); Deaths: 4,377 (31); CFR: 3.6%

Post #13: Common Sense Rules

Mar. 12, 2020

The Task Force released guidance for everyday people at a press event two days ago. Essentially the same information is repackaged into simple infographics, they provide mitigation strategies to prevent the spread of COVID-19. Apart from directing people in households with sick family members to give the sick person their own room and keep the door closed, and, advising transportation services to increase ventilation by opening windows, the advice is the same. Because of the way the virus is spread, they reiterate the universal need for vigilant hand hygiene (i.e., washing, covering cough/sneeze); regularly disinfecting high-touch surfaces; avoiding crowds and nonessential travel; food handling precautions (i.e., don't share food or utensils); and stay at home if you're sick. Not surprisingly, a new alert warned, "Stop handshaking –use other non-contact methods of greeting." Heeding this, the NBA arrested their season, and the NCAA March Madness basketball tournament will be played without fans. Still, Pence insists that he and Trump will continue shaking hands. They say, "common sense is not so common." So, there's your proof.

Cases: 127,767 (1,282); Deaths: 4,718 (37); CFR: 3.7%

Post #14: Hunkering Down

Mar. 14, 2020

It's difficult to find bottled water; folks are hoarding TP, and hand sanitizer flew off the shelves weeks ago. My parents (in their 70s) made one final pilgrimage to COSTCO before pledging to stay home until this blows over. I haven't experienced an apocalyptic vibe like this since Y2K. The US is now #8 on the leader board for cases, colleges are canceling in-classroom instruction, public schools are closing, and states have begun locking down "hot zones" with high rates of community spread. Where's this all headed and how do we prepare? I've long had the prognosis that it's going to get worse before it gets better. Experts agree. My best guesstimate is 4-6 weeks before rates begin to dampen, given our epidemic curve (i.e., # of new cases/day) and patterns shown in other countries so far. Authorities recommend that families create a household plan of action. Stock 2-weeks supply of medications, food, and essentials; have childcare plans if forced to telework; plan to take care of vulnerable family members; create an emergency contact list and establish ways to communicate with others. My family has a Zoom call scheduled for today.

Cases: 146,676 (2,195); Deaths: 5,533 (49); CFR: 3.8%

Post #15: Solace in Spirituality

Mar. 15, 2020

It's Sunday morning and I'm choosing to view church service online. Add congregating for worship to the growing list of freedoms loss (both self-imposed and recommended) due to COVID-19. I'm not quarantined, but it sure feels like it. For those who are, it's often unpleasant. Separation from loved ones, the loss of freedom, uncertainty over disease status, sadness, and boredom can create dramatic effects. Those working remotely may miss the personal interaction with co-workers and must fight simply "dialing it in." Self-imposers may go unrecognized for their altruism. Yet, it's precisely those kinds of sacrifices that are needed to squash a pandemic. During times like this, it might do us well to recharge spiritually. I'm not referring to religion here, but spirituality, "the quality of being concerned with the human spirit or soul as opposed to material or physical things." In Italy, a country with 60 million in quarantine, residents serenade each other by signing out of the windows to fight the loneliness and boost morale. They remind us that some things can't be locked down (music, laughter, self-reflection, hope). This too shall pass.

Cases: 156,881 (2,808); Deaths: 5,762 (59); CFR: 3.7%

Post #16: Viral Bigotry

Mar. 16, 2020

Fear of the unknown leads to the stigma which can lead to bigotry. We saw it with Ebola (Africans), SARS (Asians), MERS (Arabs), even as far back as 1853 with yellow fever (European immigrants). Oddly, there's been a sort of "reverse bigotry" as some claim that blacks don't get it. Ah, the harms of tribalism. It doesn't help that our leaders continue to play the blame game, deflecting responsibility for their clumsy response to the pandemic, while engaging in self-congratulatory "happy talk" that did little to prepare the public for the threat. Xenophobia has been a consistent tenet of the current administration. But as a country, we're better than that. This is a time for fact-based solidarity. Facts first. The virus did originate in Wuhan, China, but is not called the Wuhan virus. COVID-19 is not a disease "carried" by Asians. You can't "catch it" by eating Chinese food. And, no, black people aren't innately immune. The virus does not recognize borders. Likewise, it should be evident to everyone that the virus doesn't discriminate. Like social distancing, it's the collective responsibility of us all to spread facts, not hate.

Cases: 167,103 (3,599); Deaths: 6,329 (66); CFR: 3.8%

Post #17: Betting on Coronavirus

Mar. 18, 2020

Two days ago, President Trump said the coronavirus could last through July or August. That was a mistake. A pandemic is no time for speculation. It's wiser to say, "We don't know." Because we don't. This is a NEW virus with no established pattern of seasonality. There's no evidence that it will die off with warmer weather. What we do know, is that cases continue to rise; due partly to expanded testing, partly to more spread. We have not yet reached the peak of our "epi-curve." Until cases peak, then begin to dampen, no one can forecast with any accuracy when this will end. Some suggest we look to South Korea. They argue that because we're a few weeks behind them our course might be like theirs. I say we can't expect to BE where they are unless we're prepared to DO what they did. They've been far more aggressive than us, locking down cities, disinfecting public spaces, drive-through testing points, etc. What can be said with 100% certainty is our course will depend upon our collective response (i.e., practice social distancing, self-quarantine, isolation, and flu hygiene). Trump is betting on coronavirus. I'm betting on us.

Cases: 203,727 (7,048); Deaths: 8,218 (116); CFR: 4.0%

Post #18: Young Invincibles

Mar. 19, 2020

It's spring break time. Despite the urging by government officials to practice social distancing, young people pack beaches and bars determined to party come hell or high-water. Such is the mentality of the "young invincibles," a term made popular during the rollout of Obamacare to describe those who were unlikely to purchase health insurance because they didn't believe they'd need it. Now, faced with a pandemic, and amid lower death rates among those under 30 years old, college coeds tempt the odds of contracting the novel virus and transmitting it to those who are at-risk for serious complications. They say, "We're just living for the moment." I get it. It sucks to make plans and spend money only to have'em threatened by a pandemic. That's inconvenient. But perhaps a longer-term view is in order. We're learning that young people aren't altogether spared. Many in Italy have become critically ill. What's more, if we don't flatten our curve, we will run out of hospital and ICU beds before long. Of course, this will increase preventable deaths for ALL ages. We're in crisis mode, folks. It's time to be a grown-up, not a vector.

Cases: 234,000 (11,810); Deaths: 9,800 (179); CFR: 4.2%

Post #19: Stockouts

Mar. 21, 2020

Some health workers are forced to use a single mask all day then recycle it or use a homemade type. This results in personal risk to them, their families, and patients, potentially increasing person-to-person spread. How'd we get here? Even with the best contingency planning, there's seldom enough "stuff" to go around during times of extreme demand. What's critical, however, is the speed at which predictable shortfalls can be met by "flipping the switch" on pre-established protocols and surge capacity. It's March and it feels like our government is just starting to plan. One week bringing together retail pharmacies, enlisting 3M and Honeywell to mass-produce masks the next. The following week tapping emergency stockpiles. A week later, invoking the Defense Production Act to increase the supply of protective gear, and so on. In truth, we should have activated contingency plans when we learned about the impending threat in December. Ben Franklin once said, "If you fail to plan, you are planning to fail." He was right. If only we had a global health security unit to help thwart such threats early. Oh, that's right, Trump dismantled it.

Cases: 262,900 (17,836); Deaths: 11,159 (238); CFR: 4.2%

Post #20: Celebrity Roll Call

Mar. 23, 2020

I remember when Magic announced his retirement from basketball because he contracted HIV. Celebrities like Katie Couric (cancer), Toni Braxton (lupus), and Michael J. Fox (Parkinson's) have each been linked to diseases, electing to help humanize the ailments, raise awareness, combat stigma, and model resilience. COVID-19 presents the same opportunity as famous people begin to emerge as unexpected role models. Infected notables include actors Tom Hanks and Idris Elba, Bravo's talk show host Andy Cohen, NBA superstar Kevin Durant (Nets), NFL coach Sean Payton (Saints), legendary opera singer Placido Domingo, and others. More will be added to the list in the following weeks and months. Some celebrities struggle to find a role during this public health crisis leading them to act out. For example, one publicly denounced social distancing in the name of freedom (Um, the freedom to infect others?), and flaunted her kids as "gymnastic vectors." Thankfully, most celebs choose to be responsible. When they do, their sacrifice, adherence to safety guidelines, and optimism demonstrate that if they can do it, we can do it.

Cases: 328,500 (32,722); Deaths: 14,496 (416); CFR: 4.4%

Post #21: Big-Ups

Mar. 24, 2020

It feels like an episode of the Twilight Zone called "Opposite Day." Cases are going up, almost exponentially. Deaths increased by more than 200 in the past 24 hours. We're now 3rd in the world behind only China and Italy. Yet, against his own social distancing guidelines, Trump can't resist giving high-fives... to himself. At every press briefing, he pushes pass experts, bureaucrats, and sycophants at the crowded podium to give HIMSELF kudos on the terrific job he's doing in the war against coronavirus. He closed borders, sent out millions of test kits, invoked the Defense Production Act, most recently directing the Army Corps of Engineers to build hospitals in NYC. Indeed, thanks to him, millions of articles of PPE are en route this very moment. Best of all, stocks soared today in response to the $2 trillion stimulus package, the "biggest in American history." When asked, Trump graded himself a 10 out of 10 for his response. Now he's predicting the end of the scourge by Easter—less than 3 weeks away! Talk about doubling down. There's a real discrepancy here between facts and fantasy. Let's save the "big-ups" for when the cases go down.

Cases: 406,900 (52,215); Deaths: 18,293 (675); CFR: 4.5%

Post #22: Money, Money, Money

Mar. 29, 2020

As we fast approach the end of the 15-day national social distancing period, with Easter looming, Trump signed the bipartisan $2 trillion economic rescue package. I'd take a well-executed pandemic preparedness plan over a package, but that ship sailed a while ago. So, where's the money going? There are several beneficiaries. Large corporations affected (e.g., the hospitality industry) can access $500 billion. On the other end, everyday Americans who earn less than $75K/year will get $1,200/mo. (plus $500 per child). Between these two extremes are large allocations for small businesses ($377B) and our overwhelmed health care system ($150B). There's money earmarked for state and local governments, unemployment benefits, and tax breaks to incentivize companies that don't lay off workers. The CARES Act, as it is dubbed, is basically a combination of the biggest corporate bailout package ever, much-needed aid for our besieged health system, with a few time-limited sweeteners for small businesses and folks trying to make ends meet. Lawmakers contend the money will buoy our tanking economy. Let's hope they're right.

Cases: 696,900 (135,738); Deaths: 33,261 (2,391); CFR: 4.8%

Post #23: Surge!

Mar. 31, 2020

Anticipating a surge is a part of pandemic planning. Strategies to manage the dramatic influx of patients focus on rapidly creating additional capacity to meet the excess demand. Suddenly, points of care are in frantic need of more space, more staff, and more stuff. This often translates into surge tents, a call to volunteers and retirees, and rationing. We hear horror stories about the lack of PPE with increasing regularity. How doctors and nurses brave the contagion for long shifts with only makeshift or recycled protective gear between them and the virus. We've seen and heard the bleak testimonies from terrified nurses describing war zone conditions, patients dying alone, and pop-up morgues in the form of refrigerated trucks. Desperate, some care providers are forced to share disinfected goggles with other hospital staff. I met a nurse online that epitomized this plight. Her reddened face bore a rash in the shape of an N95 respirator, she told of how she isolates herself from her husband and child, fearing the worst. What I told her I would tell all the frontline heroes, "Thank you. Bless you. Hope is here. Help is on the way."

Cases: 815,100 (173,741); Deaths: 40,237 (3,433); CFR: 4.9%

Post #24: Bogus Rx

Apr. 1, 2020

"There is no proven safe and effective direct therapy for coronavirus disease." Dr. Fauci said that on Mar. 26. It wasn't his first time. Despite warnings, fraudulent claims abound. Some tout drugs that are approved for other conditions, like malaria (hydroxychloroquine). But such anecdotal reports do not meet the scientific rigor required to ensure that the medicine used for COVID-19 is effective and safe if used "off-label" for compassionate or investigational reasons. Several bogus cures have been debunked. These include garlic, chlorine bleach, sesame oil nasal spray, and silver solution. I understand that anti-COVID-19 medications seem slow in coming. I also appreciate grappling with the fear of the unknown or a need to take control. This cabin fever is making us all bonkers! But let's keep it together people. It's true, certain supplements (e.g., vit. C, zinc, garlic) can boost your immune system. But that's not a cure. When at your wit's end to find an antidote, here's a few 3-letter acronyms that I'd recommend you turn to: WHO, CDC, and FDA. If the latest concoction is not greenlit by all three, it's best that you pass on it.

Cases: 868,100 (188,247); Deaths: 43,010 (3,921); CFR: 5.0%

Post #25: Invisible Enemy?

Apr. 5, 2020

America accounts for nearly a third of the world's cases. Our epi-curve continues to go straight up as we shelter in place bracing for the worst weeks yet. The task force predicts that we'll lose up to 200,000 lives. Meanwhile, Trump poses a question that no one has asked, "What if we did nothing?" he ponders out loud. "It would be closer to 2 million deaths." Er, OK. I didn't know doing nothing was an option. Our wartime president reminds us constantly about the "invisible enemy" that we never saw coming. Yet, he continues to slow-walk the response. Top of mind for him is the fact that he's #1 on Facebook or has "Superbowl-like ratings." Unwilling to step off stage even momentarily, he obstructs the screen during the slide presentation poised to reclaim the podium and answer technical questions to our collective chagrin. Why? Grandiose sense of self-importance? A need for constant praise and admiration? A sense of entitlement? Yes. These (along with 'Exploits others without guilt or shame; and 'Frequently demeans, intimidates, bullies, or belittles others') are textbook signs of narcissistic personality disorder. Not so invisible.

Cases: 1.2M (336,619); Deaths: 68K (9,631); CFR: 5.7%

Post #26: Cover Up

Apr. 6, 2020

During a recent briefing, Trump said, "Most people could just make something out of a certain material." The next day, CDC published a new cloth face-covering recommendation. Soon after, the Surgeon General released a DIY video showing how to make one with a piece of fabric and two rubber bands. Based on the new guidelines "A cloth face covering is not intended to protect the wearer, but it may prevent the spread of the virus from the wearer to others." This seems logical. But where's the science to back this? Dr. Adams "unpacked" the reasoning behind this latest pivot explaining that the initial recommendations to avoid wearing masks were based on "the best evidence available at the time." But "we now know that a significant portion of people infected with coronavirus lack symptoms." Huh? We've known for months that 80% of infected people have little or no symptoms. This is suspect. Coronavirus policy should be informed by science. If officials start distorting/repurposing science to fit the fanciful notions of unqualified leaders, we're heading down a slippery slope. Confusing the message is one thing. Propaganda is something else altogether.

Cases: 1.3M (365K); Deaths: 73K (11K); CFR: 5.6%

Post #27: Celebrity Roll Call Too

Apr. 8, 2020

During the dark days of the coronavirus, pandemic hours drag on like days and days feel like weeks. Boredom from the confines of my apartment suspends time in a way that not even Netflix can quicken. Only 2 weeks ago I posted "Celebrity Roll Call' (Mar. 23) to show that the virus doesn't discriminate and to highlight celebrity role models that were taking the disease seriously by responsibly self-quarantining. Predictably, there've been additional infections among the rich and famous. These include Chris Cuomo (CNN), Boris Johnson (UK Prime Minister), Prince Charles (of Wales), Senator Rand Paul (R-KY), Pink & Sara Bareilles (singers), James Dolan (Owner, NY Knicks), and many others. Not so predictable, however, was the steep escalation in cases. Then, we had roughly 33,000 cases and 400 deaths. Today, we lead all countries with nearly 400,000 and have the third most deaths (behind Italy & Spain) with roughly 13,000. What a difference 2 weeks can make! We still haven't peaked in terms of new infections. Social distancing (albeit painful) remains the most effective strategy to dampen the impact and speed a return to normalcy.

Cases: 1.4M (398K); Deaths: 83K (13K); CFR: 5.9%

Post #28: Race Matters

Apr. 9, 2020

"When white America has a cold, black America has the flu." This long-held adage has been validated by decades of statistics. The health of blacks is worse across nearly every health indicator from preventable hospitalizations to life expectancy. The causes are both simple and complicated. Simple because it's obvious that those with less health insurance, income, employment, education, stable housing, internet access, health literacy, etc. have poorer health outcomes. Complicated because many of these social determinants are rooted in prejudice, racism, and social injustice. Moreover, unequal medical treatment (another important factor) reflects deeply seeded innate biases. Albeit troubling, it's not surprising that in places like Chicago, NYC, Milwaukee, and Louisiana more blacks & Latinos have died from COVID-19 than others, likely reflecting higher rates of pre-existing conditions (e.g., hypertension), delayed presentation to the hospital, off-target messaging, varying use of face coverings, or a combination. COVID-19 has exposed many chinks in the armor of our dis-ease care system. Tackling these in the post-pandemic period would be heroic.

Cases: 1.4M (430K); Deaths: 89K (15K); CFR: 6.4%

Post #29: Easter

Apr. 12, 2020

Dear Pastor,

The pandemic has caused excessive loss and suffering. The world has 1.7 million confirmed cases and 100,000 COVID-19 deaths. Sadly, the US leads the world in both cases and deaths. People are strained mentally and spiritually in ways unimaginable. But they sacrifice despite the boredom, financial uncertainty, and lack of human contact in order to decrease spread and hasten the end of this plague. Despite social distancing laws, some clergy have insisted on congregating to worship in-person. Recently, a pastor in Tampa, FL was arrested for holding church service against public orders. A Cincinnati churchgoer said, "I wouldn't be anywhere else. I'm covered in Jesus' blood," when asked about the risk to herself and others. Another declared, "The blood of Jesus cures every disease. Psalms 91. Read it." Life looks different nowadays. Easter worship should too. The Vatican shut down its traditional mass in St. Peter's Square in observance of the coronavirus lockdown. Instead, Pope Francis broadcasted service. There is sanctuary beyond buildings and hope devoid of assembly. Preach, preacher. Just do so remotely, online.

Signed,
Data

Cases: 1.7M (530K); Deaths: 111K (21K); CFR: 6.5%

Post #30: Déjà vu

Apr. 17, 2020

Have you ever shouted at the screen during the climax of a movie? You know, the scene when the villain seems subdued or dead and the protagonist turns her back. The music crescendos and then it happens. The villain summons one last gasp of energy to attack the hero who has let down her guard, feeling triumphant. I hope this scenario does not happen when it comes to reopening the economy. We are dealing with a formidable enemy. It has outwitted our response to date, killing more than 31,000. It has a remarkably high attack rate and lays dormant in millions of people who are without symptoms or test results. We lack a vaccine, effective therapeutics, and adequate testing; not to mention ongoing shortages of PPE, contact tracing foot soldiers, and surge capacity for the second wave of infections on the heels of this current wave. Novel viruses often have multiple waves. Like most, I have an unquenchable thirst to get to our new normal. I applaud the science-informed phased approach outlined by the feds, but I remain cautiously optimistic that we are not dropping our guard prematurely. We have all seen this movie before. It does not always end well.

Cases: 2.1M (673K); Deaths: 145K (31K); CFR: 6.9%

Post #31: Coping

Apr. 20, 2020

Ironically, staying at home is wearing me out. I was introverted and worked from home before the pandemic. Still, I find these restrictions mentally draining. It took a few weeks to burn out on CNN. Apparently, every story is "breaking news." The fitness room in my building is closed, leaving me with my ankle weights, a foam roller, and a yoga mat. The rooftop deck: closed. The club room: closed. The university tracks: closed. That makes it tough for me as a club coach and hurdler. My hamstrings rejoice. I stretch, do 7-minute ab workouts, and calisthenics. It feels a bit like middle school P.E. To fight cabin fever, I walk or jog a 2-mile loop in my neighborhood a few times a week. The best part is my weekly trip to the grocery store. Most of my day is spent banging away on my laptop, reading, watching news online, and writing. The balance is spent on Zoom, calls, preparing meals, and eating. Is anyone else tired of cooking? Like the lyric in the Talking Heads song, "same as it ever was," each day bleeds into the next. Sure, I have my list of personal projects, but the fatigue of monotony leaves me with little energy to start them.

Cases: 2.4M (780K); Deaths: 165K (38K); CFR: 6.9%

Post #32: Trumptastic

Apr. 24, 2020

During a call-in radio show a week ago a caller asked me about rubbing alcohol: If alcohol killed the virus on hard surfaces and worked in hand sanitizer, "Why couldn't we make an inhaler, like for asthma, and use it to kill the virus in our lungs?" I replied, "Your instincts make sense. But the problem here is a matter of safety and efficacy." I explained that isopropyl alcohol could be toxic, causing airways to shut down (bronchospasm) causing a bad asthma attack, even death. If perfumes, tobacco smoke, and pollen can trigger asthma, imagine what aerosolized alcohol could do, I said. I appreciated his question as a layperson with pedestrian science knowledge and zero medical training. I'd expect more if he were surrounded by the nation's top docs and scientists, you know, like our president. The latest barrage of Trumptastic questions from the podium—not at a planning meeting, or debriefing—was about the internal use of disinfectants like Clorox and Lysol. Really? Injecting disinfectants? He came short of saying, "What have you got to lose?" as he did about the unproven hydroxychloroquine. Your life, Mr. President. You can lose your life.

Cases: 2.6M (867K); Deaths: 185K (45K); CFR: 7.1%

Post #33: Double Whammy

Apr. 26, 2020

Last week, Dr. Redfield, CDC Director, became the subject of controversy after saying, "There's a possibility that the assault of the virus on our nation next winter will be even more difficult ..." Today, our healthcare system is still reeling from the surge of patients with COVID-19. Imagine if both the seasonal flu and the novel coronavirus hit at the same time. This double whammy could paralyze our hospitals, resulting in all-time highs of flu-like illnesses and deaths. The fortunate fact is that flu season (which typically peaks between December & February) was ending when our first case of community-acquired COVID-19 was confirmed on February 26. Luckily, we avoided the perfect storm. Of course, Trump attempted to make Dr. Redfield recant his commonsense statement. Instead, he timidly paraphrased his warning, then admitted he was "accurately quoted" earlier. Truth-telling shouldn't be an act of defiance. I'm in favor of "injecting" the American people with the truth. There has been plenty of talk about bleach and Lysol lately, but sunlight is the best disinfectant. Willful ignorance only increases the death tolls unnecessarily.

Cases: 2.9M (939K); Deaths: 198K (48K); CFR: 6.8%

Post #34: Mo' Money

Apr. 26, 2020

How much will it cost to get us through this pandemic? A few days ago, Congress passed, and Trump signed into law, the 4th economic stimulus package. Following $2.2 trillion last month, this brings the total to $3 trillion. And more will be needed. This time around, most of the money ($370 billion) is earmarked for small business loans, grants, and paycheck protection. With record numbers of Americans filing for unemployment, some receiving food bank handouts for the first time, this is crucial. The previous money ran out quickly, partly because big public companies (e.g., Ruth's Chris Steakhouse, Potbelly, and Shake Shack) laid claims to some of those funds. Some volunteered to give the money back. Others will face stiff penalties if they do not. Of the remaining money, $75 billion will go to prop up overwhelmed hospitals, and $25 billion is allotted to expanding testing. Sub-optimal testing for COVID-19 has been the Achilles heel of our country's response. Yet, having adequate testing is one of the keys to allowing people to safely return to work. Perhaps better oversight will ensure both the dollars and tests are distributed equitably.

Cases: 2.9M (965K); Deaths: 200K (50K); CFR: 6.9%

Post #35: Family Ties

Apr. 28, 2020

Social distancing may be a misnomer. Many have suggested using the term "physical distancing" instead. I agree. A silver lining of this pandemic for me has been (re)connecting with family. So far, through the power of Zoom, I have joined a half dozen such calls. These calls have been part well checks, part reunion. On Easter, I counted 23 screens on my laptop. Last weekend I spoke with cousins for the first time in decades. I heard the good news that my niece was accepted at LSU and about my 2nd cousin's prestigious internship at the Academy of Television Arts & Science. I received updates from those working essential jobs, those adapting to working from home, furloughed, back in school, and retired. We even looped in my younger brother who lives in Germany. These real-time updates are priceless. Family defines us. It strengthens & sustains us. I know it seems cliché to say, "We're all in this together." But like it or not, we are. And when it comes to family, regardless of how you define it, checking in and visually confirming the wellbeing of loved ones is like chicken soup for the soul. Hopefully, this ritual will be part of the new normal.

Cases: 3M (990K); Deaths: 205K (51K); CFR: 6.8%

Post #36: Vaccine Uptake

Apr. 30, 2020

Most Americans vaguely remember the last pandemic. It was the H1N1 pandemic of 2009. Also called Swine flu, this novel flu virus threatened to disrupt life as we knew it. There were school dismissals, antiviral medications tested, vaccines developed, & eventually, FDA approved for use. President Obama even proclaimed National Influenza Vaccination Week (Jan. 2010), encouraging all Americans to observe the week by getting vaccinated with the 2009 H1N1 flu vaccine. If only Americans were so eager. The uptake of the vaccine was only about 33%. When the dust settled, there were 60 million cases and 12,500 deaths from H1N1. Today, rates of people receiving the seasonal flu vaccine remain low. Only 4 in 10 reports receiving the vaccine (which includes protection from H1N1). Seniors do the best (6 in 10) and adults between 18 – 49 years do the worse (3 in 10). Not terrific. As bogus treatments (i.e., disinfectants, Hydroxychloroquine) are debunked, America holds out for a vaccine to defeat COVID-19. But there's little evidence that they will line up to get it when it arrives. Looks like we better keep washing our hands & covering our coughs.

Cases: 3.1M (1.1M); Deaths: 230K (62K); CFR: 7.4%

Post #37: Reopening Right

May 2, 2020

There is a saying among carpenters, "Measure twice, cut once." This literally means measure carefully to avoid making a mistake requiring the need to cut again, wasting time and wood. This proverb applies to COVID-19. Admittedly, reopening the economy is part science—that is, based on the cases, deaths, ICU bed usage, ventilator use, etc.—and part gamble because predictive models based on the epi-curve are not 100%. They are, well, predictive. As of May 1, nearly two dozen states have begun to reopen. Georgia started earliest on April 24th. Most states are proceeding with caution while others seem almost random. For example, I might question prioritizing reopening gyms, hair and nail salons, barbershops, and massage parlors. In Illinois, where I live, we shifted to a modified stay-at-home order through May; Chicago may extend it through June. Prudent. Most experts believe that reopening the economy should occur only after ensuring that rapid diagnostic tests are available in every community. I agree. But in the interim, let's keep measuring (monitoring the COVID-19 data) even as we modify guidance to safely reopen albeit gradually.

Cases: 3.3M (1.1M); Deaths: 242K (66K); CFR: 7.3%

Post #38: What's Good?

May 5, 2020

The pandemic has not been managed well. Still, the curve is flattening, the death toll may be less than estimated (100 – 200K), and states have begun to reopen. I want to highlight some of the positives. Without commentary, the top 5 things that have gone right are … #5. Assembling a task force to provide scientific, policy, and economic advice. #4. Issuing national guidelines to slow the spread of coronavirus, including stay-at-home guidance which most states mandated. #3. Opening diagnostic testing beyond CDC and public health labs. #2. State coalitions to coordinate a regional approach to reopening economies amid White House posturing. #1. Dr. Anthony Fauci. C'mon, this guy is a national treasure and probably the only advisor who gives straight talk to America (and Trump). Now, a few honorable mentions: $25B in the last relief package to boost testing; Trump's activation of the Defense Production Act, albeit underutilized (testing supplies & PPE); SBA funding for small business paycheck protection (although insufficient oversight, allowing the LA Lakers, Shake Shack, & others to siphon funds). It's been a bumpy ride, but we're getting there.

Cases: 3.5M (1.2M); Deaths: 252K (70K); CFR: 7.2%

Post #39: Collateral Damage

May 11, 2020

As with every new virus, outbreak, epidemic, and pandemic, we continue to learn lessons during the activity. The novel coronavirus is no exception. We have learned this virus is more contagious than initially thought and can be transmitted from those without symptoms. It's more deadly than the flu by a factor of 20x. And not only does it wreak havoc on your lungs (the primary site of illness), but it causes other strange symptoms seemingly unrelated to the respiratory system. For example, it can cause damage to the kidney, heart, brain, even the toes. Let's discuss this. Early on, patients noticed a change in taste & smell. More recently, there's been an increase in dialysis, strokes, & heart attacks mostly due to blood clots. Clots also occur in small blood vessels in the fingers and toes, causing "COVID toes." The virus attacks men more than women, the old more than the young, and the obese more than those of normal body weight. Fortunately, to date, the virus does not complicate pregnancy as with the recent Zika virus. The mystery of COVID-19 is still unfolding. So far, the virus has taught us much and school is still in session.

Cases: 4M (1.3M); Deaths: 283K (80K); CFR: 7.1%

Post #40: Guinea pig-in-chief

May 18, 2020

Why would anyone want to take a medication meant for one condition for a completely different condition that they do not even have? That would be like taking an aspirin to prevent from getting a sinus infection. Who does that? Apparently, the leader of the free world, that's who. Today, Trump boastfully announced that he's been taking, wait for it… hydroxychloroquine for a week, even though he does not have COVID-19. The medical and scientific community warns against its side effects, including life-threatening heart problems. And there is no proof that it works to cure, speed recovery, or prevent the COVID-19 which, again, Trump does not have. If he did, he would know immediately because he is tested regularly. His FDA advises against its use unless enrolled in a clinical study and under the supervision of a physician. Yet Trump has decided to go rogue. As usual, no one in his political or social orbits would dare convince him otherwise. That Trump would risk his health to make the point that his genius rivals that of doctors & scientists is pure folly. That he would put others at risk by his bad example is disgraceful.

Cases: 4.7M (1.5M); Deaths: 318K (90K); CFR: 6.8%

Post #41: Death Rate Controversy

May 24, 2020

How deadly is coronavirus? Is the death rate 1% based on opinion (making it 10x as deadly as the seasonal flu)? Or is it closer to the calculated 6% based on actual data (math check: 96K/1.6M x 100 = 6%)? The answer is both. You see, when an epidemic is unfolding, there are lots of assumptions, models, & estimates. These constantly change. Often, it is not until the dust has settled and the data is "cleaned" do we reconcile our best understanding of the epidemiologic truth. Likely the number of deaths has been undercounted so far because people died early during the flu season from COVID-19, and many died outside of the healthcare system, but were not counted. Moreover, there are far more cases of COVID-19 than the 1.6M count would suggest. Many cases had mild or no symptoms or did not meet the criteria to receive a test given tests shortages. Therefore, they remain undiagnosed. The bottom line, expanding testing would help tremendously, but it's not an exact science. My educated guesstimate is that the final death rate will fall between 1% – 2%. That's still 10x – 20x higher than the flu. Until then, we use the numbers we have.

Cases: 5.2M (1.6M); Deaths: 342K (97K); CFR: 6.6%

Post #42: Donald Is No Duck

May 25, 2020

It could be argued that Americans have excess. Our poor still live better than most of the world despite the economic downturn. It is hard to deny our nation's relative embarrassment of riches. Ironically, it is our deficit that has led to our undoing during this historic moment. Not the deficit of test kits, ventilators, health workers, or even PPE. I am referring to the most painfully obvious deficit: leadership. The buck stops at the top, always. Trump muzzles scientists, distort facts and fakes a new area of expertise every week. So bankrupt as a leader that he lacks transparency, diplomacy, empathy, humility, integrity, and accountability, qualities essential for leadership. Clearly, the deficit of accurate, consistent, information emanates from the White House. As we near 100,000 deaths, imagine our country's response to this pandemic under President (fill in the blank), republican or democrat. How many tens of thousands of lives would have been spared? This is not a partisan issue. They say, if it looks like a duck, swims like a duck, & quacks like a duck, then it is probably a duck. As far as leadership goes, this Donald is no duck.

Cases: 5.4M (1.6M); Deaths: 345K (98K); CFR: 6.4%

Post #43: Are We There Yet?

May 29, 2020

We surpassed 100,000 deaths and are rapidly closing in on 2 million cases (an underestimate!). How close are we to achieving herd immunity? Herd immunity (or herd protection) occurs when 70-80 percent of a population has immunity to novel coronavirus. This happens if they were infected, or if they received an effective vaccine for the bug. To meet this threshold, more than 230 million Americans would need to become immune to protect the remaining 100 million. Assuming 20% of infected people are symptomatic and 80% are without symptoms and therefore would not have been tested, we MAY have reached a population immunity of 10% (rough estimate). That's about 30 million people. So, when it comes to herd immunity, we are not there yet. Sure, the person-to-person spread will continue, fortunately, slower because of physical distancing & the widespread use of masks, but it will take a vaccine to get us the rest of the way, if possible. Sweden employed a herd immunity strategy with lax precautions, allowing social gatherings. Not only is this risky given the fatality rate of this virus, but it has not worked. They have only achieved about 7% immunity.

Cases: 5.8M (1.8M); Deaths: 364K (103K); CFR: 6.3%

Total COVID-19 deaths in the U.S. through May 2020

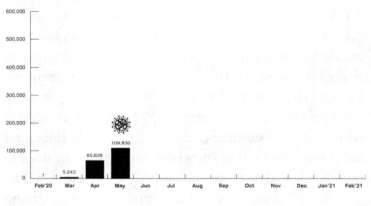

Source: Worldometer

PART 2: SUMMER MADNESS

The uptick in cases following Memorial Day foretold a pattern that would be consistent throughout the pandemic. Cases rose after each holiday. Simply put, Americans found it difficult to curb social norms. Summer became the period of resolute denial leading to more hotspots around the country. COVID fatigue combined with the lure of summer cookouts, family gatherings, and kids home from school, proved stronger than the need to maintain social distance and wearing masks consistently. I shared my thoughts about the importance of observing public health measures while returning to normal activities in an article by USA Today.

The easing of social distancing restrictions by many states led to increasing case counts. By June 10, the US had reached 2 million cases. As Operation Warp Speed hummed along in search of viable vaccine candidates, hydroxychloroquine, the miracle drug hyped by Trump, was debunked. In early July, we learned that coronavirus could be airborne. This news led to heightened concerns about the risks posed by indoor crowding, including workplaces and schools. Thankfully, several vaccine candidates (e.g., Moderna, AstraZeneca) began to show promising results.

As COVID-19 climbed to the third leading cause of death in the US (after heart disease and cancer) by mid-August, it was clear that more financial relief would be needed. In late July, the US Senate introduced the second round of stimulus: the Health, Economic Assistance, Liability Protection, and Schools (HEALS) Act. Unfortunately, talks between the White House and Democrats stalled despite soaring unemployment rates leaving the vulnerable among us—people of color, low-income, and workers deemed essential—to fend for themselves as best they could. Despite the numbers (or perhaps because of them), our President insisted that the origin of increased cases was increased testing. Emboldened by this belief, Trump repeatedly hosted superspreading events.

In the midst of the summer swelter, two camps of freedom fighters emerged. There were those fighting for their right to be exposed (and expose others) to a phony virus by returning to work and refusing to wear facemasks or take precautions. Many were stoked by politicians eager to reopen the economy. More poignantly, there was also mounting civil unrest protesting police brutality in the aftermath of the May 25th murder of George Floyd that was sparked in the US and spread around the globe.

During a CNN interview, I was asked about the risks to demonstrators posed by the mass gatherings for criminal justice reform. My answer: context matters. Every day people do a personal risk assessment in navigating how best to meet their daily needs. Using the framework of Maslow's hierarchy of needs, I said that as needs go, "human rights and breathing are right at the top of the list," implying that the magnitude of their cause might justify the risk. Disaggregating the contribution of these mass gatherings from those related to states' premature re-openings and widespread noncompliance with safety precautions would be impossible, I stated.

Post #44: Perfect Storm

June 9, 2020

States are showing daily highs of up to 1,000 new cases. With the perfect storm, this could've been predicted. First, states were reopening for weeks (with various degrees of caution). Second, many relaxed precautions for the Memorial Day holiday. Fed up with being inside for months, many were quick to throw social distancing out the window in favor of barbecues and fun in the sun. Third, in the aftermath of the murder of George Floyd by members of the Minneapolis PD, tens of thousands took to the streets in protest of the death and the larger issue of persistent police brutality against black men and communities of color. Many protesting wear face coverings, however, physical distancing is not being practiced. Fourth, nationwide testing has increased dramatically, thus diagnosing more cases. The exact contribution of protests to the spikes in cases is unknown. Indeed, protesters are making an informed, calculated, assessment, fully understanding their personal risk. We take risks for milk & eggs, gasoline, exercise, and essential jobs. Doing so for human rights is not only reasonable, for many it is obligatory.

Cases: 7.1M (2M); Deaths: 411K (112K); CFR: 5.8%

Post #45: Don't Shoot the Messenger, Please

June 18, 2020

When it comes to the pandemic, too often public health officials are being blamed. But they did not create COVID-19. Their job involves tracking and interpreting the numbers, following guidance, and informing elected officials (mayors, county executives, & governors) how to proceed in a way that best safeguards the health of the people they are charged to protect. I know because I've been the top health official for a county (NY) and state (IL), and led the organization that supports the nation's 3,000 local health departments. Health officials use the best available scientific information to inform their recommendations. But the final call is made by the elected official. The current targeting of public health leaders is unprecedented and dangerous. Reportedly, 27 local and state officials have been forced out since April due to pressure, scapegoating, and an angry public. We are all frustrated with lockdowns and a stalled economy. But the real enemy is the virus, not public servants who aim to protect the public from the virus. Blaming the bearer of bad news for being responsible for that bad news is pointless.

Cases: 8.3M (2.2M); Deaths: 450K (118K); CFR: 5.4%

Post #46: Social "Dissing"

June 19, 2020

People seem less friendly nowadays. I wonder if this is a sign of frustration due to lockdowns and face masks. We, humans, hate to be inconvenienced. Still, I would have expected the agitation to fade with the reopening of the economy. When this began (in March), it seemed that every person was for themselves, hoarding TP, cleaning products, and water. Then things calmed down a bit. Now, with the widespread use of masks, only the top half of a stranger's face is visible. But so often I am met with angry eyes, nods, or exaggerated gestures. People shop with their heads down. Like robots, they walk up and down grocery store aisles and through checkout lines in virtual silence. It is almost as if they think being stealth and refusing to acknowledge others will stop the transmission of the virus. You can smile with your eyes. You can wave with your eyebrows, or, better yet, your hands. Social distancing should not equate to "social dissing." During these tense times, I pray we graduate from acts of selfishness and demonstrate more patience and kindness. COVID-19 has forced us to sacrifice much. Good manners should not be among the casualties.

Cases: 8.4M (2.2M); Deaths: 454K (119K); CFR: 5.4%

Post #47: False Equivalence

June 26, 2020

There is a serious problem brewing. More than half of the states have seen a rebound in COVID-19 cases over recent days and weeks. Some have posted their highest numbers since April. Texas and California all reported more than 5,000 new cases each. Florida and Oklahoma had record single-day highs. And in Arizona, hospitalizations continue to peak while ICUs quickly fill. What is the problem? There has been a false equivalence. Many residents mistakenly believe that reopening has signaled the "all clear." It has not. The reopening was made possible because collectively we changed our behaviors (e.g., social distancing, sheltering in place, and wearing masks). That led to flattening the epidemic curve and easing pressure on our healthcare systems. Unfortunately, we are going in the reverse direction now. Some states have responded by pausing further reopening. Others have made masks mandatory in public. Still, others choose to ignore the obvious. This ain't rocket science. It's epidemiology. We MUST follow the numbers. When will we learn to dance with the one who brought us?

Cases: 9.5M (2.4M); Deaths: 488K (124K); CFR: 5.1%

Post #48: Attention Pregnant Women

June 28, 2020

As with many aspects of this pandemic (e.g., face masks, therapies, flattening the curve), the situation is evolving. As the science changes, the recommendations to the public should change. The latest science shows that pregnant women are at higher risk of complications from COVID-19. Here is what we know. Compared to nonpregnant women with COVID-19, pregnant women with COVID-19 are 440% more likely to require hospitalizations; 50% more likely to be admitted to ICUs; and 70% more likely to need a ventilator. According to the CDC study, Asian women, & those between the age of 35 – 44 years were at higher risks. Fortunately, there was no difference in death rates between the two groups. We have known for some time that the virus attacks men more than women, the old more than the young, the obese more than those of normal body weight, and those with some preexisting conditions. Add pregnant women to the high-risk list. Science is not perfect. It can take time. However, it beats conjecture every day and twice on Sundays. The key to beating COVID-19 is our ability to pivot with humility. When we know better, we got to do better.

Cases: 9.9M (2.5M); Deaths: 499K (125K); CFR: 5.0%

Post #49: Pricey Proposition

July 1, 2020

It happened with insulin and the opioid overdose drug, naloxone. Now, the anti-viral Remdesivir. Some call it price gouging. Others call it sound business. The fact is, Gilead, the maker of Remdesivir, received $100 million in taxpayers' support to develop it. Now that it has been shown to shorten hospitalization of COVID-19 patients by 4 days, they're charging up to $3,120 for the treatment. Apparently, they factored into their price the savings from a shorter hospital stay, avoiding a costly ICU bed, and the greater societal good of potentially fewer infectious patients in the community. But thus far, the drug has NOT shown improvement in death rates. Is this pricing fair given that we are in the worse economic downturn in modern history, and the uneven burden of disease on those who can least afford it? U.S. healthcare cost is exorbitant. But hospitals, health system stewards, and big pharma often say, "there can be no mission without margin." I get it. But in this case, where's the public's return on their investment? Sadly, the affordability of medicines is a persistent reason why our healthcare system remains broken.

Cases: 10.5M (2.7M); Deaths: 513K (128K); CFR: 4.9%

Post #50: Unmasked Maverick

July 2, 2020

When did protecting your personal and family health become so controversial? How did we get to the place where exposing others to a very contagious infection (albeit often asymptomatic) is a constitutional right? After some initial confusion about masks, the White House promoted cloth coverings as a theoretical barrier of protection. Later, science endorsed this behavior showing that it can reduce transmission of the coronavirus by up to 50%. States incorporated masks into their reopening plans. News reporters, elected officials, essential workers, and the man on the street don face covers, responsibly. Yet, our maverick-in-chief refuses to do so. Wisely, Trump's inner circle, party sycophants, even his VP (sometimes) wear masks. Instead of following his task force guidance, Trump's on the campaign trail whipping naked-faced rally-goers into a lather at packed rallies. Even as WH aids and secret service members contract the disease (presumably at his rallies!), Trump simply "can't see himself wearing one." Clearly, the message from our Commander in Chief to supporters is "do as I do, not as I say." So much for leading by example.

Cases: 10.8M (2.8M); Deaths: 518K (129K); CFR: 4.8%

Post #51: Independence Day?

July 4, 2020

Experts warned us during spring break. But young students, feeling invincible, "just wanted to live." Warnings were issued for Memorial Day weekend. But many were cooped up for far too long to heed the warning. Then there were the protesters. Not those marching for policing reforms. Those storming capitals to protest their rights to work amidst the wide community spread of the virus. Some were even asserting their right to risk their own lives, holding signs that read "give me liberty or give me COVID-19!" Eventually, the anti-stay-at-home rallies withered as states began reopening. What followed these displays of freedom was a predictable & precipitous rise in cases, especially among the younger groups. The curve is no longer flat, it is sloping upward. Indeed, independence is about freedom of expression, peaceful assembly, and the right to petition the government. But should these rights allow citizens to freely if unwittingly, put their neighbor's health at risk? Patriotism should spark us to behave in ways that protect our fellow Americans. The freedom of a few, should never imperil the lives of the many. Let's make America SAFE again.

Cases: 11M (2.8M); Deaths: 526K (130K); CFR: 4.9%

Post #52: Problem Well Stated

July 8, 2020

There are more than 3 million diagnosed COVID-19 cases in the U.S. That's a disproportional 25% of the world's total. Yet, there's no sign of that warm weather miracle as promised, you know, where "the virus just disappears." The 3 million number equates to roughly 5 times that number (15 million) because 80% of infected people are asymptomatic (and presumably not tested). That's nearly 5 percent of the nation's population. Furthermore, in a recent Washington Post survey, 13% of all U.S. adults said they know someone who has died from COVID-19. For blacks & Latinos, the percentages reported were 31% and 17%, respectively. These disproportionate experiences reinforce what the data has shown from the beginning: racial and ethnic minorities are hit hardest by the virus, facing higher hospitalization and death rates. Those who study social determinants of health know the story well. But it was refreshing to hear Dr. Fauci during a recent House Oversight Committee articulate the "double whammy" of preexisting chronic diseases and institutional racism. As the saying goes, "a problem well stated, is a problem half solved."

Cases: 11.9M (3M); Deaths: 548K (132K); CFR: 4.6%

Post #53: Corona Goes Airborne?

July 12, 2020

From the onset of the pandemic, we have known that coronavirus is a respiratory virus. It attacks our airways (from mouth & nose to lungs), replicates there, and spews out from our airways when we cough, sneeze or even speak. When it does, virus-containing droplets can travel through the air up to 6 feet before landing on a surface, somewhere. So, what's all the hubbub (i.e., scientists petitioning the WHO to upgrade the status of the virus to an airborne one) about the virus being airborne? Simply put, while heavy droplets land in 6 feet, fine respiratory mist (or aerosol) can linger in the air longer. Absent a strong cross breeze or a robust ventilation system to dilute the concentration of the virus-containing mist, the risk of infection is much higher. That said, what must we do differently to remain safe? 1) Be diligent about wearing masks & social distancing, 2) Avoid crowded indoor environments for prolonged periods, and 3) if concerned, ask about the HEPA air filtration systems of public institutions, including schools, businesses, nursing homes, places of worship. The science is not definitive, but better safe than sorry.

Cases: 12.7M (3.2M); Deaths: 565K (135K); CFR: 4.4%

Post #54: Holy Stitt!

July 16, 2020

The coronavirus caught up with another brash-talking elected official. I watched Gov. Stitt at the Trump rally in Tulsa last month. You know the one attended by an unmasked, smaller than anticipated, frenzied crowd. Then, Gov. Kevin Stitt, 48, led the cheers and scoffed at the idea of wearing face coverings. Now he is the first Governor to test positive for COVID-19. Worst yet, his state has surging rates of new infections. In fact, over the past few weeks, Oklahoma has posted its highest numbers of new cases, and 7-day averages, since the beginning of the pandemic. There's always a lag between exposure and clinical symptoms. We call that the incubation period. Clearly, the rally helped fuel the statewide uptick in cases and is likely where Gov. Stitt was exposed. This is not a "gotcha moment" so much as it is a cautionary tale. Politics aside, to paraphrase a popular superhero TV show I watched growing up, it proves that this SUPER-virus is "Faster than a speeding reopening! More powerful than a GOP loyalist! Able to leap tall denials at a single bound!" I wish Gov. Stitt has a speedy recovery and a fresh perspective going forward.

Cases: 13.7M (3.6M); Deaths: 588K (138K); CFR: 4.3%

Post #55: School Daze

July 18, 2020

When schools reopen in a month, it may be a case of "one step forward, two steps back." I say this because Israel tried to reopen schools in May. Slowly at first, with small groups & staggered classes. Then they lifted restrictions. Two weeks later they shut them down after COVID outbreaks in kindergartens, middle schools, and high schools. More than 200 students & a dozen teachers got infected. Nearly 7,000 were mandated to home quarantine. Some schools were spared, but the hysteria of "what if" prompted many parents to yank their students out of the classrooms, opting for remote learning. Similar school-based outbreaks occurred in Singapore & S. Korea, two countries that managed the pandemic far better than us. Surprisingly, the White House balked at CDC's school guidance, stating it was "too tough." Education Secretary DeVos conceded there's no national playbook to safely reopen schools. She suggests schools simply figure it out. Plans will likely include in-person, remote-only, and hybrid models. None of these would work if teachers were too sick to teach. Let's hope this experiment doesn't devolve into a futile game of "hokey-pokey."

Cases: 14.1M (3.7M); Deaths: 599K (140K); CFR: 4.2%

Post #56: Mickey Can Wait

July 23, 2020

Some of my most cherished memories as a kid were made at the magic kingdom. I grew up in southern California, so I visited Disneyland located near Los Angeles. Back then we purchased a book of color-coded Disney coupons that we used for rides, attractions, and food. A lot has changed since then. Nowadays things are done digitally. The admission price (albeit a small fortune for a family) entitles you to all the rides. But much has not changed, including the crowds and long lines at popular rides, busy food courts, and gift shops. No doubt about it, the kingdom is an interactive, almost communal, extremely high-touch, place. Social distancing all but defeats the purpose. So why would Disney World in Orlando, FL re-open? COVID cases are sharply increasing nationwide, and Florida is the epicenter of the global crisis. Even with temperature checks at entry & constantly disinfecting surfaces, it defies all rational thinking. I can't imagine what's more discouraging, Disney's attempt to salvage summer revenue or exhausted parents traumatized by home-schooling duties, and faced with a sparsity of summer activities for their kids. I wish all those who brave the turn-styles the healing power of pixie dust.

Cases: 15.2M (3.9M); Deaths: 623K (143K); CFR: 4.1%

Post #57: Lifeline Threatened

July 30, 2020

As of May, roughly 20 million Americans are without jobs. This pandemic recession equates to an unemployment rate of 16%. This falls somewhere between rates during the 2007 Great Recession (13%) & the Great Depression of the 1930s (25%). Adding insult to economic injury, the stimulus program (CARES Act) that topped-up weekly unemployment benefits by $600 for those eligible, and extended state benefits to a max of 39 weeks, are set to end on July 31. Um, that's tomorrow. Without this lifeline, those struggling to make ends meet due to no fault of their own will suffer mightily. A political tug-a-war pits a liberal-minded House against a suspiciously-frugal Senate, the former advocating to extend current relief through the calendar year, the latter wanting to decrease payments to $200, then drop it to equal 70% of an individual's salary when combined with the state's unemployment. Evidently, the Senate is worried that the present stimulus will deter people from returning to work. With our economy on life support, states re-closing, & consumer confidence shot; it's difficult to envision an economic recovery if consumers have no income.

Cases: 16.9M (4.4M); Deaths: 667K (151K); CFR: 3.9%

Post #58: Back to School Spoiler Alert

Aug. 8, 2020

A picture is worth a thousand words. But at the risk of sounding like a soothsayer or Captain Obvious, I will proceed with a synopsis of Georgia. They reopened their economy early, then saw a cosmic rebound in cases. More recently, the Governor sued the Mayor of Atlanta for requiring face masks and limiting the size of public gatherings. Last week, they were one of the first states to send students back to school. Spoiler alert, if the first week is a predictor of what's to come, this in-person back-to-school experiment doesn't end well. High-schoolers were all smiles & a few masks as they packed hallways. Masks are not required in Georgia, merely recommended. Is it surprising that most students opted to not wear them? The early results are in for Cherokee County, Ga. Symptoms and positive tests for COVID-19 among students and teachers has led to 260 students and 8 teachers being quarantine. The school added an online choice, but the majority of students plan to return on Monday, masks optional. The school district superintendent admitted that the photo "does not look good." Um, now who's sounding like Captain Obvious?

Cases: 18.3M (5M); Deaths: 694K (162K); CFR: 3.8%

Post #59: Hydroxy Misinformation

Aug. 10, 2020

True, hydroxychloroquine has a long track record for treating medical conditions (i.e., malaria, rheumatoid arthritis). But it does not work for COVID-19. The latest ambassador for false hype is a newly formed, partisan, America's Frontline Doctors. Their pro-hydroxy campaign was personified by the Houston-based, Nigerian, physician Dr. Immanuel. Flanked by other physicians, she went viral on the strength of Trump's retweet. However, within hours the video was removed from Twitter & other social media for sharing false information. Shortly thereafter, the Texas Medical Board warned physicians against making false claims about COVID cures. Facts: there are no FDA-approved drugs to prevent or treat COVID-19. For months, the NIH has warned against using hydroxy for the virus. Despite several rigorous studies, hydroxy proved ineffective (and potentially harmful) even when combining with zinc & azithromycin. I ardently support physicians sharing their experiences. We all have our biases. As a physician & former CDC disease detective, mine leans towards strong evidence. Free speech? Absolutely. Fake facts? No thank you. There is a difference between anecdotes and science.

Cases: 19.8M (5M); Deaths: 738K (162K); CFR: 3.7%

Post #60: Mask Up Fam!

Aug. 25, 2020

Early on some blacks believed we were "immune" to "the Rona." It is now widely known (based on infection and death rates) that minorities are hardest hit by the virus. Thankfully, as science trickles in, most sensible people change their minds AND their behaviors. The science on masks has evolved too. There is no denying that they are protective. Yet, mask-wearing has not been done consistently by many, including those in vulnerable communities of color. Disturbingly, frequent media reports appear about house parties in cities like Chicago, Atlanta, and elsewhere attended by swarms of people that disregard the threat of COVID-19. No masks. No social distancing. No worries? Ahem, there is a disconnect if our most vulnerable are the least protected due to willful recklessness. This ain't a resource problem. A good reusable mask costs less than $10. It's a crisis communication problem and let's be real an accountability problem. Minorities will benefit from culturally relevant risk mitigation messaging by credible messengers. But we also need to level up and be more responsible. Mask up fam! We can't afford to ignore life-saving commonsense measures.

Cases: 26.3M (5.7M); Deaths: 813K (177K); CFR: 3.1%

Post #61: Some Masks Don't Work

Aug. 25, 2020

All masks are not created equal. Early in the pandemic, we were warned by experts to keep our hands off the medical-grade masks. It's best to leave those for the frontline health workers. Then we were told that any face covering would do. DIY videos began appearing and suddenly wearing bandanas was in style. People began using industrial masks, and masks with changeable filters, and valved masks. A recent study by scientists from Duke's physics department showed that some masks don't work very well. Some even make matters worse! Using a simple laser set-up to visualize and measure droplets expressed when people talk, the findings showed that the fitted N95 masks were the most effective. No surprise there. Three-layer surgical masks and homemade cotton masks also work well. Folded bandanas and knit fabric masks performed poorly. And worst of all neck fleeces (called gaiter masks) & masks with exhalation valves. These split respiratory droplets into smaller more airborne, micro-droplets, thus increasing the risk for transmitting the virus. Bottom line: face masks save lives. However, all masks aren't created equal. Avoid gaiters, knit fabric, and bandanas.

Cases: 26.3M (5.8M); Deaths: 815K (178K); CFR: 3.1%

Post #62: Superspreading on the White House Lawn?

Aug. 28, 2020

2,000 guests attended the RNC finale last evening on the south lawn of the People's House. Perhaps missed by the casual observer, I noted an unwelcomed guest in attendance as well: the novel coronavirus. And due to the conduct of denial—shaking hands, sitting shoulder to shoulder, and, well, socializing... it was spreading! 90% didn't wear masks. None practiced social distancing. It was the kind of crowd that states have prohibited for months as a pandemic mitigation strategy. It's too soon to know for sure, but this had all of the trappings of a superspreading event, one in which a few infected people infect many. The program lasted hours. And with the notable exception of the venue being outdoors, we've seen how this can end. We've seen rapid transmission among crowds at the Trump rally in Tulsa (attended by the late Herman Cain) a few months ago, packed hallways at reopened schools, corporate conferences. For the optimistically delusional, the gathering may have signaled an end to the COVID crisis and a return to normalcy. For the woke, the display was a harbinger of trouble & a reminder that things will continue to get worse before they get better.

Cases: 24.4M (5.8); Deaths: 832K (181K); CFR: 3.4%

Total COVID-19 deaths in the U.S. through August 2020

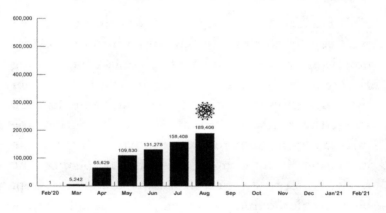

Source: Worldometer

PART 3: FALL BACKWARDS

Guidance continued to change with the evolving science during the fall. In addition to several promising vaccine candidates that are fast approaching Emergency Use Authorization by the FDA, other therapies show potential. Most Americans learned about these new treatments when Trump became infected with the coronavirus in early October. He was hospitalized for three days. While hospitalized, he received every treatment available, well everything except hydroxychloroquine. Out of an abundance of caution, he was given the antiviral remdesivir, dexamethasone (a steroid), and an investigational antibody cocktail called Regeneron. His recovery was uneventful.

Upon his return to the White House, Trump remained deviant about wearing a face mask. His leading by bad example was not lost on the scientific community. In an article published in a prestigious medical journal, 34 editors criticized him (and other leaders) for "turning a crisis into a tragedy." Disregarding the guidance from the scientific community, and his own Coronavirus Task Force, Trump sponsored and attended a number of super spreader events. One such event that took place at Rose Garden resulted in nearly three dozen infections, including White House staff.

Mixed messages from our political leaders, particularly those in red states, no doubt fueled the rise in transmission rates. Cases continued to spike and on November 4, the US reported an unprecedented 100,000 cases in a single day. The nation braced itself for the impact of seasonal flu cases on top of escalating COVID-19 cases and the resultant strain on the healthcare system stretched to the brink. A national study confirmed what I described in an op-ed published in the Chicago Tribune, stating that Americans, especially those younger than 65 years, aren't great at getting their flu shot. The study recorded the national flu vaccination rate at only 52% overall, with even lower rates among Blacks and Latinos. Unfortunately, the pandemic would continue to expose racial and ethnic disparities in healthcare, and the issue of vaccine hesitancy among people of color.

Post #63: Convalescent Plasma

Sept. 1, 2020

Remarkably, our body's system of white blood cells can quickly kill bugs that it has seen before and fight them off. It has the memory to mount a response and attack them before they become a problem. There are two basic ways to achieve this immunity. The most common, called "active immunity" occurs either through infection with the novel coronavirus, for example, or after you've been vaccinated for COVID. In both cases, it takes a few weeks for our body's immune system to rev up. There is no vaccine for COVID yet, and scientists are unclear about how long those previously infected are immune. The other way to gain immunity is called "passive immunity." As the term implies, antibodies present in the blood (convalescent plasma) of people who've recovered from COVID is "passively" infused into sick patients. Theoretically, this MAY immediately boost one's ability to fight the virus. That's why the FDA has authorized its emergency use for hospitalized patients. However, there's no solid evidence that it's safe or works to treat COVID-19. In fact, the NIH's treatment guideline panel recommends against this at this time.

Cases: 25.5M (6M); Deaths: 852K (184K); CFR: 3.3%

Post #64: COVID on Campus

Sept. 3, 2020

More than 1,000 students at the University of Alabama tested positive for coronavirus within 2 weeks of returning. I'm a parent and I'm worried. I have 3 daughters at large universities. They've been back for 4 weeks. They are mainly schooling remotely, with clubs and extracurriculars occurring via Zoom. One's in a residence hall, two reside in apartment communities that cater heavily to college students. My youngest, an athlete at a Power Five conference school, was tested upon returning to campus. She's negative, but her former in-person-turned-virtual study partner tested positive, lost her sense of taste and smell, and is in a 14-day quarantine. My other daughters were given facemasks and lots of safety information when they returned. Undoubtedly, like other students, my daughters' courageous spirits have been dampened by fear and cautionary tales. I warn them to be responsible & forego big social clusters, but also to avoid self-imprisonment. "Mask up and go out every day and walk, exercise, get a dose of sunshine and fresh air," I say. And if given a choice between hybrid & distance learning at a professor's discretion, "choose distance for now."

Cases: 26M (6.1M); Deaths: 863K (186K); CFR: 3.3%

Post #65: Summer Sadness

Sept. 7, 2020

As Americans, we savor our long weekends. Perhaps because we're so overworked with too few vacation days, we tend to go all out. The bookends of summer are Memorial Day (signals the start) and Labor Day which marks its end. For each holiday, plus Independence Day, we seem to shift to a recreational mindset, making big plans to reward ourselves with barbeques, beach parties, and other social gatherings. It's all good, normally. But due to COVID-19, things haven't been normal for a minute. The consistent guidance has been to wash our hands often, keep gatherings small, wear masks, social distance, and keep it brief. Sadly, the holiday attitude prevailed. This has led to many planning/attending crowded outdoor children's parties, park grillings, backyards, and bars, often without masks. In other words, not much has changed except for the COVID tally. There were huge spikes in cases & deaths after these holidays. As of Memorial Day, the virus had claimed 98,000 lives. Today (Labor Day), that death toll is roughly 190,000. That's nearly 100,000 dead in 3 months! There's plenty of blame to go around for this devastation. The sobering fact is that we must fault ourselves as well.

Cases: 26M (6.2M); Deaths: 836K (189K); CFR: 3.2%

Post #66: Celebrity Roll Call III

Sept. 15, 2020

The coronavirus does not discriminate. Not by political party affiliation, race, or celebrity status. Although we've restarted our economy, resumed major sports (albeit in a bubble absent of crowds), the precautionary guidance has not changed much. Predictably, since my second post on this subject (April 8), more celebs have tested positive, despite preexisting conditions and many doing all the right things. Notables include funny men (Kevin Hart & D.L. Hughley), news anchors (Brooke Baldwin & George Stephanopoulos), a housewife (Jennifer Aydin), the walking dead (actor Michael Rooker), and those breaking bad (actor Bryan Cranston), even a Doja Cat. There was a bevy of actors (Alyssa Milano, Antonio Banderas), a Babyface (Kenneth Edmonds), and royalty (singer Prince Royce and former Miss USA, Shanna Moakler). So ubiquitous is the virus that even Usain Bolt couldn't outrun it. He succumbed days after attending a maskless in-person celebration for his 34th birthday. No one can be completely insulated. But this shouldn't deter us from being responsible. When we are, we harness the best of ourselves, reduce our risk, & protect our neighbors.

Cases: 29M (6.5M); Deaths: 928K (194K); CFR: 3.2%

Post #67: Trump and COVID-19

Oct. 3, 2020

Trump has had a precarious relationship with COVID since the onset of the pandemic. Today, you cannot say Trump without saying (or thinking) COVID. The two unwitting bedfellows will be forever linked. What began in February with denials, magical promises, and self-congratulating pats on the back, morphed into botched responses replete with disinfectant, UV light, hydroxychloroquine, a war against masks, hijacking scientific data, and muzzling voices of scientific reason at "warp speed." And now reportedly the virus has caught up with the commander in chief, despite regularly testing those around him. Is this surprising given the dozens of rallies he's held and the fact that several of his staff contracted the virus during the pandemic? Real scientists have said that no one is without risk. They've warned that despite most being asymptomatic, those at high risk for complications are over age 60, obese, & with other health conditions. President Trump checks these boxes. I join the nation in wishing Trump well. I pray too for a wake-up call to our nation: coronavirus is ubiquitous, relentless, and undaunted by fictional bubbles or bluster.

Cases: 34.6M (7.3M); Deaths: 1M (208K); CFR: 2.9%

Post #68: COVID Presidential Playbook

Oct. 4, 2020

For 8 months, the country learned mitigation strategies for coronavirus. Yet, despite 7M cases and over 200-thousand deaths in the US, the pandemic was more of a theoretical threat than a real one for many. Some even called it fake. Until now. With Trump's diagnosis, the response playbook for COVID-19 is on national display. It's the same 3 steps experts have preached from the onset: 1) Risk assessment. He's a high risk given his age, obesity, and most likely has chronic diseases (e.g., prediabetes, hypertension). 2) Symptoms review. If absent or mild, a 14-day quarantine would be sufficient. Trump's moderate symptoms required oxygen, antiviral medication (Remdesivir), & hospitalization. Immune-boosting antibodies are usually reserved for the most severe symptoms on a "compassionate use" basis, but Trump received that too. 3) Contact tracing. In addition to

Melania & his senior aid Hope Hicks, those testing positive (so far!) include Kellyanne Conway, Trump's campaign manager Bill Stepien, a hand full of senators, and the president of Notre Dame University (with apologies). As it turns out, COVID is no conspiracy, and science does matter.

Cases: 34.9M (7.4M); Deaths: 1M (209K); CFR: 2.9%

Post #69: Roll Call: Executive Branch Edition

Oct. 5, 2020

There's a reason experts recommend a 14-day quarantine. Recall, that the incubation period—the time from infection to showing symptoms—is 2 to 14 days. It can also take days for tests to detect the virus. Of course, most people don't have symptoms. So, for those who had close contact with the President, it may be wise to test again at the end of their quarantine, regardless. Reports have been inconsistent about when Trump first tested positive. Was he a super spreader or simply the sponsor of many superspreading events? We may never know. We can, however, expect his web of contacts to continue to expand for the next 2 weeks, with more high-profile names being added to the list. Those COVID-positive include the Republican National Committee chair Ronna McDaniel, senators Mike Lee (UT), Thom Tillis (NC), Ron Johnson (WI), and Ex-NJ Governor Chris Christie. Those testing negative include other members of the Trump family, VP Pence & his wife, VP Biden & Sen. Harris, cabinet secretaries Azar (Health), Pompeo (State), Mnuchin (Treasury), Bar (AG). Also, Supreme Court nominee Amy Coney Barrett is in the clear. But we still have 10 more days of watchful waiting.

Cases: 34.9M (7.4M); Deaths: 1M (209K); CFR: 2.9%

Post #70: Presidential Pomposity!

Oct. 17, 2020

Trump contracted the virus due to his recklessness and rejection of scientific guidelines. He balked at face coverings for himself AND discouraged others from protecting themselves as a partisan show of loyalty. He poo-pooed guidance from his administration's health and research agencies. He ignored social distancing rules by repeatedly sponsoring unmasked super spreader events on the White House lawn. The latest event resulted in dozens getting the virus and national security threat, even as contact tracing is ongoing. Hospitalized and treated by a team of doctors, he was given everything but the kitchen sink, including an experimental medicine reserved for those critically ill and requiring a ventilator. Once released from the hospital—after taking a spin in the motorcade, likely infecting his driver and security detail—he rips off his mask the first chance he gets. Not long after, he tweets 'Don't be afraid of COVID. Don't let it dominate your life.' Remarkable. He received a level of care that no one else is entitled to, survives, then tweets 'don't be afraid.' Indeed, a mistake that makes you humble is better than a "cure" that makes you arrogant.

Cases: 36M (7.5M); Deaths: 1M (211K); CFR: 2.8%

Post #71: Risky Business

Oct. 19, 2020

With cooler temperatures upon us, and flu season nearly here, more of us will be huddling inside. Transmission of this air-borne infection increases indoors with poorer air circulation. We are all vulnerable, but especially people with underlying chronic conditions. 6 in 10 American adults meet these criteria because they have at least one chronic health condition; 42 percent of adults have two or more chronic conditions. For example, 1 in 4 have hypertension, 1 in 5 have high cholesterol, 1 in 10 have diabetes, and 1 in 18 have asthma. If you are one of these, your risk for contracting COVID doesn't change, but your risk for complications if you get it does! Dr. Fauci—the nation's top infectious disease expert—emphasized this fact in a recent presser. In response, Trump, who continues to host "super spreader" events, called him a "disaster" and an "idiot" about coronavirus. The irony is flabbergasting. There will most certainly be a second wave of infection. Each of us has a choice to make. Either follow the advice of experts based on epidemiologic evidence or follow President Trump, someone whose only credential is having been infected & infecting dozens of others.

Cases: 40M (8.1M); Deaths: 1.1M (219K); CFR: 2.8%

Post #72: Good Air Up There

Oct. 23, 2020

Hospitality industries like lodging, theme parks, and transportation, have been hit hard by imposed restrictions to slow the pandemic. Whilst cruise lines stay anchored, airlines are beginning to look up. The reason? Science. Recent studies show in-flight air filtration systems along with mandatory mask-wearing are effective in reducing potential viral transmission. Add to this enhanced sanitizing protocols, and you have a SAFER cabin environment. Estimating the number of COIVD cases linked to flying (or the precise transmission rates) can be tricky. It's tough to reproduce passenger behavior on planes and even tougher to prove that cases were infected during a flight. But there's reason to be optimistic. Barring any mile-high superspreading events, and supported by these findings, cash-strapped airlines have resumed selling all seats, instead of reserving the middle seat empty to allow a few feet between strangers. Bottom line: your risk for COVID will increase anytime you leave your personal bubble. But thanks to good air, flying seems relatively safe. I take solace in knowing there's something to be gained from the arctic blast that otherwise makes flying so uncomfortable.

Cases: 42M (8.5M); Deaths: 1.1M (224K); CFR: 2.6%

Post #73: New Pre-existing Disease

Oct. 24, 2020

We've heard a lot about pre-existing diseases because people with them are at higher risk for complications and death from COVID. Also, because the Trump White House has been trying to abolish this benefit along with the entirety of Obamacare. Ironically, COVID-19 (Trump's Achilles heel) may soon be added to the growing list of pre-existing conditions. If so, this could mean that health insurance companies and employers will start screening everyone for the infection. They don't do this for the influenza virus (seasonal flu), but coronavirus is turning out to be very different. In addition to the 10-fold higher death rate, people with the bug are hammered with organ damage that can result in lasting 'brain fog,' hypertension, irregular heartbeat, shortness of breath, even joint pain. Even those with mild disease may suffer tissue damage and scarring. Regrettably, at this point, we don't know the full spectrum of long-term problems, who's at most risk, or how to lessen the risk. Immunity after infection is great. But immunity wanes. Unfortunately, the damage from the virus lingers. All the more reason to fight to keep coverage for those with pre-existing conditions.

Cases: 42M (8.5M); Deaths: 1.1M (225K); CFR: 2.6%

Post #74: COVID Raises Deaths from All Causes

Oct. 29, 2020

With daily COVID media coverage, the average person on the street knows there's been 200,000-plus deaths and counting. But laypeople don't realize this number is an underestimate. Here's why. First, it doesn't account for every death from COVID-19. People who were never tested die undiagnosed. Some die outside of a hospital. Second, indirect deaths due to disruptions in the health care system aren't counted. For example, shortage of hospital beds prevents some with heart disease, Alzheimer's, or other conditions from getting the care they need causing their premature death. As such, the pandemic has led to increased deaths from all causes. We call this 'excess deaths' from COVID. Epidemiologists use the term to refer to deaths that would not have occurred over the same period if there wasn't a pandemic. A recent study estimates that all deaths in the US increased by 20% during COVID. Most (67%) were attributed directly to COVID, but a third were from other causes arising in the context of an overburdened health system. Whether it's measured by mental, financial, or health currency, the cost of COVID is more than meets the eye.

Cases: 44M (8.9M); Deaths: 1.1M (227K); CFR: 2.5%

Post #75: Halloween, Spooky Risky?

Oct. 30, 2020

An opportunity to dress up, show out, and rake in lots of sweet treats, Halloween has always held the specter of risk. Tainted treats, delinquent mischief, pedestrian and alcohol-related traffic accidents, spikes in theft, and vandalism are commonplace. This year, we must add COVID to the list of threats. Thankfully, we need not throw out the baby with the costume. Those who choose to do so can still enjoy the festivities while remaining safe. CDC has provided some commonsense guidelines to help. They advise making trick-or-treating safer by avoiding direct contact with trick-or-treaters, giving out treats outdoors, setting up a station with individually bagged treats for kids to take. It goes without saying that staying 6 feet away from non-family members, washing hands before handling treats, & wearing a mask (if age 2 or older) are a must. Less risky family activities include pumpkin carving, costume parades, outdoor Halloween-themed scavenger hunt, or visiting a pumpkin patch. Remember, children are not immune to COVID. Although most have no symptoms or mild disease, they still pose scary risks for transmitting the virus to older family members.

Cases: 45M (9M); Deaths: 1.1M (228K); CFR: 2.4%

Post #76: Is Testing to Blame?

Nov. 6, 2020

"We have more testing than anyone. That's why we have more cases." We've heard Trump & co. make this claim repeatedly. Testing creates COVID cases about as much as turning on the kitchen light creates roaches. They were there all along, in the dark. Testing simply illuminates what's already true. It doesn't magnify cases. It merely helps estimate the number of infections. Even still, most experts agree that case counts are actually an underestimate by at least 50% because most infected people are asymptomatic & don't seek testing. Indeed, the best way to minimize a viral pandemic is to simply not test (or undertest) for the virus. Epidemiologists call this a surveillance bias. It's the idea that the more you test, the more you find, and vice versa. By dialing down testing when community spread was obvious, Team Trump practiced this bias. Testing is now more widely available but still not equally accessible to all communities. And while testing is key, more important metrics include hospital/ICU bed usage, those on ventilators, & deaths. These are real people fighting for every breath & sometimes losing. Testing cannot be blamed for this heartbreaking reality.

Cases: 49M (9.8M); Deaths: 1.2M (236K); CFR: 2.4%

Post #77: Vaccine Nears Finish Line

Nov. 9, 2020

The pharmaceutical companies Pfizer & BioNTech are one step closer to crossing the finish line. No small feat given the competition running at "warp speed." Safety data for the vaccine candidate is still pending, but when compared to the placebo group, the 2-dose vaccine was 90% effective in preventing infection among those vaccinated. To be sure, these are encouraging results for the final phase (Phase 3) of the vaccine clinical trial. However, the "brew" is not yet shelf-ready. So far, there are 94 confirmed cases among a global study group of 43,000+ diverse participants. More information on safety & efficacy will need to be collected until the confirmed case count reaches 164, with additional safety data collected for 2 months after that. During this next period of the trial, vaccine effectiveness estimates may change, and/or safety concerns may arise. But if all goes well, the company seeks to get FDA approval for emergency use. They anticipate producing 50 million doses in 2020 & 1.3 billion doses in 2021 for global distribution. With hospitals and local economies buckling under the weight of record infections, this would be a welcomed respite.

Cases: 50M (10.1M); Deaths: 1.2M (238K); CFR: 2.4%

Post #78: Who's Up First?

Nov. 18, 2020

The saying goes, "vaccines don't help, vaccinations do." Meaning, regardless of the effectiveness of the new vaccines if people do not roll up their sleeves and get the shot it doesn't much matter. But who will be the first to get it? As with any scarce commodity, there will be rationing. States and cities continue to put together their distribution plans and logistics may be a nightmare. Suffice it to say, no plan will be identical. Each will vary based on infection rates, hospital capacity, nursing home density, economic drivers, etc. A panel of national experts recommends a general action plan based on priority groups at the highest risk. It is a phased approach. The "jumpstarters" are health workers, first responders, those with serious preexisting diseases, & nursing home residents. Phase 2 includes essential workers (incl. teachers, school staff), people in homeless shelters & jails, vulnerable seniors, and anyone with less serious chronic health conditions. Young adults & children fall to phase 3, along with other essential workers. Anyone else wanting the vaccine would be in phase 4. By knowing the group that you and your loved ones fall into can help manage expectations.

Cases: 56M (11.5M); Deaths: 1.3M (250K); CFR: 2.3%

Post #79: COVID and Mental Health

Nov. 19, 2020

For each one of the 250,000 COVID-19 deaths, there are 9 family members bereaved, according to a recent study. That is 2.2 million hurting from survival guilt, the sadness of not being able to say goodbye or attend the funeral, an inability to grieve in normal ways due to social isolation & quarantine. For many, the loss is amplified by uncertainties of employment, food security, personal finances, and the inability to worship at their church, synagogue, or mosque. It can feel as though there is no relief in sight. Our collective distress is showing up in the numbers. A CDC study found that 41% of adults surveyed reported at least one mental health condition (e.g., substance abuse, depression, anxiety, PTSD). These rates were 3 to 4 times higher than just a year ago. Sadly, serious consideration of suicide was reported by 11%. Overwhelmed frontline health workers are suffering from exhaustion while witnessing record daily losses. Children may have problems coping in an increasingly uncertain world. As we approach the holiday, let us be mindful of each other's mental health needs and, where possible, serve an extra portion of empathy and support to our neighbors.

Cases: 56M (11.6M); Deaths: 1.3M (251K); CFR: 2.3%

Post #80: COVID Relief Stalled

Nov. 25, 2020

Stimulus and enhanced unemployment checks ended in July. Since then, Congress has been bickering about another much-needed relief package. In the meantime, more Americans are suffering and many small businesses teeter on the brink of shuttering their shops for good. Guidance for businesses oscillates with COVID infection rates. As the holidays approach, transmission rates continue to peak, hospital ICUs fill, and the need for more shutdowns looms large. Economists say that without another injection of cash economic recovery will be difficult. At odds are the size ($500 B vs. $2 T), distribution (paycheck protection vs. state and city support), and timing (Trump or Biden's watch) of the funds. Now with a vaccine on the horizon, some lawmakers are poised to push for a skinny relief package, believing that the vaccine will speed up the economic bounce back. Thus far, sheltering in place has been the most powerful strategy to combat the virus. COVID fatigue is one thing. Surviving (i.e., rent, food, bills) is another thing altogether. Without a stimulus package (and soon!), the hustle to meet daily needs will take priority over compliance with COVID guidelines.

Cases: 59 M (12.6M); Deaths: 1.4M (260K); CFR: 2.4%

Post #81: Thanksgiving Chicken Soup

Nov. 26, 2020

There's been lots of precautionary advice from health experts for a safer holiday. For those choosing to gather in person, there are practical considerations. Specifically, there are three key questions you need to answer. Question 1: What is your personal risk? Age (over 55?), general health (obese? Smoker?), chronic diseases (asthma, hypertension, diabetes?), immune system (strong, compromised?). Question 2: What are the environmental risks? Huddling in your bubble or someone else's? Indoors or outdoors? Opening doors/windows, HEPA filter with AC? Question 3: What are the situational risks? Wearing masks when not eating? Sitting at separately distanced dinner tables? Buffet style (multiple people handling utensils) or is one gloved person making plates for everyone? Duration of the gathering? An hour or the entire day. Is hand sanitizer & Kleenex readily available? The fact is risk is both relative and cumulative. Despite the fact that there will likely be a bump in infections by Christmas due to the unavoidable Thanksgiving holiday transmission, sharing with family during the holidays is like chicken soup for the soul. We can still do our best to celebrate responsibly.

Cases: 60M (12.8M); Deaths: 1.4M (262K); CFR: 2.3%

Total COVID-19 deaths in the U.S. through November 2020

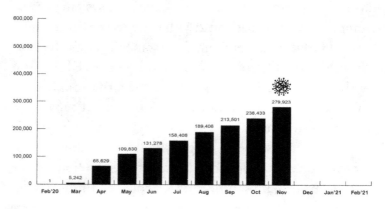

Source: Worldometer

PART 4: DARK WINTER'S LIGHT

The US continued to set record highs throughout December recording its 15 millionth case, surpassing 300,000 deaths, and hitting more than 3,000 deaths in a single day for the first time since the pandemic began. As the month ended, more than 77,000 deaths were the most of any month during the pandemic. That was a death approximately every 30 seconds for the entire month. Furthermore, the 6,427,955 new cases made it the most infectious month to date. We assumed that the cases and deaths were due to the original coronavirus. Unfortunately, as new variants of the virus were emerging in the UK and Brazil there was no way to be certain these more contagious strains weren't already here, worsening the picture.

Mercifully, with both Pfizer and Moderna vaccine candidates being awarded Emergency Use Authorization by the FDA, there was light at the end of a very dark and cold tunnel. Vaccine distribution logistics began to take shape, and priority groups for the miracle drugs were determined. According to the CDC, vaccine rollout would target health care personnel and nursing home residents first, followed by seniors, people deemed essential workers and those with serious medical conditions. Within weeks every social media feed was inundated with selfies posted by self-proclaimed heroes rolling their sleeves up to take their medicine. Profiles in courage, truly. Nonetheless, vaccination distribution proved to be a logistical challenge. While 14 million doses were distributed (not injected, distributed) to states around the county, this was well short of the set goal of 20 million by the end of the calendar year. Ultra-cold storage, poor coordination, and the lack of absorptive capacity by states to receive vaccines were largely to blame. Still, states were only using a portion of their allotments, some choosing to hold back doses.

January brought with it new leadership (Biden) and a revamped COVID task force as the US surpassed 25 million cases. That equated to one of every 13 Americans testing positive for the virus. This presented both an unprecedented challenge and an opportunity to learn from the foibles of the outgoing administration. Two such areas of need were indisputable. First, blacks and other racial/ethnic minority communities across the country were disproportionately impacted. Evidence of this included lopsided hospitalization and death rates. Given historical unequal treatment in healthcare, several measures of social vulnerability, and pre-COVID medical disparities, this could have been predicted. Second, vaccine hesitancy is unshakeable for many of these vulnerable communities.

National polls showed that the reluctance or wait-and-see posture of minorities was mainly due to concerns about safety and cutting corners to rapidly develop the vaccine. Also, for blacks, in particular, many are distrusting when it comes to what might be considered "medical experimentation" based on a legacy of racist practices. Clearly, education would be needed if the US stood any chance at all of achieving herd immunity. Along with other excerpts, I took to the media to help debunk myths about the vaccine. My series about the top 10 things Black Americans need to know about the COVID vaccine, for example, was featured in *TheGrio*, a black-owned news website reaching 6 million black Americans each month.

Post #82: Shorter Quarantining

Dec. 3, 2020

Americans are sick and tired of being sick and tired. It's called "pandemic fatigue." Given this, there's good news and bad news. The good news is that CDC has recommended shortening the self-quarantine period for those who might have been exposed to someone with COVID. The bad news is that CDC has recommended shortening the self-quarantine period for those exposed to someone with COVID. You read me right. Previously, the quarantine period was 14-days. Now CDC has relaxed the guidance allowing for a 10-day quarantine without testing, and 7 days after receiving a negative test result. In both cases, people will need to watch for symptoms for14 days after exposure. This relieves the fatigue, but I fear it may decrease adherence precisely because of the fatigue. With surging rates of new infections, the Thanksgiving free pass, and ongoing superspreading events, I doubt that shorter quarantining will help. From the onset, doing the right thing after exposure has always been about personal responsibility. Ultimately, those who are responsible will take this seriously. And those who don't... don't, regardless of the recommended duration.

Cases: 65M (14M); Deaths: 1.5M (275K); CFR: 2.3%

Post #83: Hypocrisy Risks Spread

Dec. 4, 2020

For all of his shortcomings, no one can accuse President Trump of not standing by his convictions when it comes to COVID. He believed from the start that COVID was overstated, if not a "hoax." He poo-pooed masks and social distancing and personally practiced neither. Lambasted for hosting superspreading events, he went right ahead having rallies and unmasked parties at the White House. When it came to egging on the freedom-fighting resistance, he led by example even after contracting COVID himself. That's commitment (even if misguided). The same cannot be said for the leaders who claim to take precautions seriously. Several cases of hypocrisy have come under fire. Among the high-profile cases were Governor Newsom (D-CA) dining maskless at a posh indoors restaurant during a statewide indoor dining ban, Chicago Mayor Lightfoot getting a haircut when salons were closed, and Denver Mayor Hancock seen boarding a flight to Mississippi for Thanksgiving despite urging his constituents to avoid travel and family gatherings. This pandemic requires our leaders to level up. Optics can have deadly consequences because if they don't follow their own rules, there's hardly any motivation for others to do so.

Cases: 65M (14M); Deaths: 1.5M (276K); CFR: 2.3%

Post #84: Will Vaccines be Mandatory?

Dec. 8, 2020

COVID-19 vaccines were rolled out in Russia on Saturday. Today, a 90-year-old UK woman was the first to receive the vaccine as they start their mass vaccination program. We are just a few weeks away in the U.S. The FDA will approve two vaccines for emergency use any day now. When they do, priority groups like frontline health workers can start rolling up their sleeves. But will the vaccine be mandatory? It depends. Usually, local governments (or employers) make the rules. So, when it comes to school-aged kids & college students, some vaccinations (or proof of antibodies) are required for enrollment. Likewise, high-touch, high-risk, jobs (e.g., healthcare, nursing home, food handling) require proof of certain vaccinations like hepatitis B, chickenpox. However, many states have exemptions for medical, religious, or philosophical reasons. Once FDA-approved for wide distribution and there's enough to go around, schools & some jobs may mandate the vaccine. I wouldn't expect this requirement for students until 2022. It may take that long to vaccinate all high-risk adults and to complete safety and effectiveness testing for those under age 18 years.

Cases: 68M (15M); Deaths: 1.5M (284K); CFR: 2.2%

Post #85: Blacks Remain Reluctant

Dec. 10, 2020

National surveys about the COVID-19 vaccine have been consistent. As a Black community, we are not feeling it. To be clear, skepticism is high for all Americans. However, compared to 37% of Latinos, and 56% of whites, only 27% of Blacks plan to get vaccinated. There are historical reasons for such skepticism. We hold in our DNA and collective memory scars from medical experimentation, unethical abuse, and unequal treatment. Consequently, there is no reason to expect us to roll up our sleeves and run to the front of the line for a vaccine with barely a few months of safety data. Still, we could benefit from arguably the most important medical discovery in decades, a safe and effective COVID vaccine. How do we turn the corner? In a word, education. Fear and distrust can be offset with transparency, facts, and inclusion. In this regard, both the message and messenger matter. When given reliable information from credible sources, Blacks are empowered to confidently make informed decisions about their health. Trustworthiness before trust.

Ultimately, the goal is not to sell the community (on the vaccine or anything else), it is to serve the community.

Cases: 68.9M (15M); Deaths: 1.5M (289K); CFR: 2.2%

Post #86: FDA Greenlights First Vaccine

Dec. 12, 2020

After reviewing Pfizer's data on efficacy and safety, the FDA has approved their COVID vaccine on an emergency use basis. Emergency Use Authorization (EUA) is not the same as an FDA-approved or "cleared vaccine" status. However, the vaccine meets enough criteria to show the benefits outweigh the risks. Due to alarming COVID infection/death rates & no alternatives, EUA was given. Next, CDC will give recommendations for use and priority groups, including for special populations such as youth under age 16 years, pregnant or breastfeeding women, and those with allergies within the next few days. Each state's vaccination priority plan may differ slightly, but healthcare workers and residents/staff at senior facilities will likely be first. Don't expect to find the vaccine at your local CVS or Walgreens immediately. The vaccine is in short supply and states will receive their allotment based on their population size. If you think you meet the criteria for the vaccine, discuss your options with your healthcare provider. Remember, to finish what you start. You must return 3 weeks later for a second shot to get the full benefit of the vaccine.

Cases: 68.9M (16M); Deaths: 1.5M (296K); CFR: 2.2%

Post #87: Remember Hydroxy?

Dec. 14, 2020

With so much buzz about a vaccine, many have forgotten hydroxychloroquine. Once hyped by our outgoing president as a miracle drug, he infamously asked, "What have you got to lose?" Trump later reported that he took the drug for a week. The FDA authorized it for emergency use, then amid concerns about heart problems, revoked the EUA in June. There was the fervent endorsement from a group of Houston physicians that Trump echoed and retweeted. Twitter promptly removed the content for being suspect. I wrote five previous posts on hydroxy. I herein want to put this matter to bed. A recent study involving diverse patients from 34 US hospitals compared hydroxy with placebo. Results were consistent with those found in the studies from the UK & Brazil: hydroxy did not significantly improve clinical status. According to the US study, overall survival wasn't any worse with hydroxy, but those treated with it were 2.5 times more likely to have cardiac arrest treated with CPR. Bottom line: hydroxychloroquine DOES NOT work for hospitalized adults with COVID-19. Remdesivir & corticosteroids are useful. Hydroxy, on the other hand, should be reserved for lupus & rheumatoid arthritis.

Cases: 71M (16M); Deaths: 1.6M (299K); CFR: 2.3%

Post #88: New Sheriff in Town

Dec. 15, 2020

The Electoral College has affirmed President-elect Biden's win. Now, let's begin healing. Biden named his COVID advisory team weeks ago. He asked Fauci to stay on as his chief medical advisor and brought back Dr. Rick Bright, former director of BARDA, the HHS agency that develops vaccines. Bright was ousted for "whistleblowing" about Trump's pandemic shenanigans, predicting that his snubbing of science would cost American lives. He was right. Both men deserve to be on the Biden COVID team because they told the president & American people what they needed to hear, not what they wanted to hear. They put scientific & personal integrity above politics and petty-minded self-interests. They didn't drink the bleach. Others shielded Trump's non-science babble and played poker face as he spewed absurdities about injecting UV light & disinfectants. Most lacked courage and integrity when we needed it most. Shockingly, Dr. Birx, the current COVID coordinator, wants to stay on. To clean up this mess Biden must clean house with few exemptions. The inaction of previous advisors enabled the mishandling of the pandemic. There's a new Sheriff in town. It's time to turn the page.

Cases: 72M (16.5M); Deaths: 1.6M (301K); CFR: 2.2%

Post #89: We Don't Need A Hero

Dec. 17, 2020

Unless you've been "unplugged," you have seen the media coverage of hospital workers receiving the new COVID vaccine. The scene looks the same. There's a hospital banner in the background. Cameras document the moment. Sleeve up. Shot given. Applause. Reporter interview. The attention borders on coverage for acts of heroism. I join my healthcare peers in being hopeful that a safe & effective vaccine signals the beginning of the end of the pandemic. But receiving it is hardly an act of valor. In fact, it may soon be required for most high-risk jobs like healthcare & nursing homes. Rolling up your sleeve is vital. But no more so than consistently wearing masks & social distancing. People who choose to be vaccinated are no more valiant than those who are disciplined about quarantining & hand washing. Whether you're at the front or back of the line for the shot, or if you make an informed decision to avoid it altogether, each of us is expected to meet the moment. We don't need heroes or rogue actors. We just need plain everyday folk to care enough about their fellow man to act responsibly. Let's stop exalting folks (and ourselves) for doing what is right.

Cases: 73M (17.2M); Deaths: 1.6M (310K); CFR: 2.2%

Post #90: COVID Toolbelt

Dec. 22, 2020

As our hospitals pass the breaking point, states resume lockdowns, and elected officials roll up their sleeves to inspire us to do the same, it's a good time to review the tools in the 'ol COVID Toolbelt. We have come a long way in the past 10-plus months. Guided by the evolving science and the public health epidemic playbook, here's the inventory of tools: 1) general/crisis communication, 2) handwashing & flu hygiene, 3) social distancing, 4) administrative orders (e.g., stay at home), 5) face coverings, initially reserved for health workers 6) Remdesivir (an emergency use antiviral injection given over 5 days to shorten illness), 7) antibody-containing convalescent plasma from COVID patients, 8) Regeneron (the emergency use antibody "cocktail" infusion received by Trump, Carson, Christie, and few others), 9 & 10) the Pfizer and Moderna vaccines, immune-inducing liquid gold, each requiring 2 shots separated by 4 weeks. Whew! That's some set of tools. Still, there's nothing among them that will cure COVID. Your best bet is to fiercely defend against it as if your life depended on it. Hospital beds being scarce. There's no guarantee you'll get one.

Cases: 77M (18M); Deaths: 1.7M (319K); CFR: 2.2

Post #91: New Strain Emerges!

Dec. 24, 2020

It's called antigenic drift. That's when a virus undergoes random genetic changes (called mutations) over time. Call it survival of the fittest, this clever coronavirus has begun the process of "shapeshifting." A new strain has popped up in the UK and other countries. This was predictable. Problem #1: the new strain is more contagious, although not necessarily more deadly. Problem #2: the new vaccines weren't developed for this strain. So, if (when?) this new, more infectious, strain becomes widespread, the shoulder shots heard 'round the world over the past week will be less valuable. You see, the active immunity gained from vaccination is specific for a particular virus, not all strains/types. An exact match between vaccine and virus is required for maximum protection. Although some vaccines give "cross-protection" for other strains, this is typically limited. We see this each year with seasonal flu. We anticipate 80% protection, but due to antigenic drift protection is roughly 50%. Bottom line: manufacturers will need to tweak (reformulate) their vaccines for them to be effective against emerging strains. All the more reason to remain hypervigilant with the other precautions.

Cases: 78M (18.5M); Deaths: 1.7M (326K); CFR: 2.2%

Post #92: Every 30 Seconds

Jan. 7, 2021

In the span of 30 seconds, you could text your mom, change your Facebook status, order a meal, watch a funny Superbowl halftime TV ad, or sprint a half-lap around the track. Sadly, during December, it was the average time for a COVID death, every 33 seconds to be precise. The death tally totaled more than 77,400, twice the number in November! With so many deaths, it is not surprising that more than 100,000 people were hospitalized daily for the entire month. That was another record. Real infections, real people dying, coast to coast without sparing any area of the country. The main contributing factors for the surge were the ongoing COVID fatigue, the new more contagious strain of the virus, and, of course, the holiday laxity. Together, they led to these predictable post-season swells which maybe still peaking. Unfortunately, the slow rollout of the vaccines failed to neutralize the increased deaths. Now, with our darkest days yet, and growing reports of vaccine hesitancy, the central question is: How will local, state, and federal governments revise their COVID response playbooks to help stop the carnage? Continuing the present course, costing a life every 30 seconds, is untenable.

Cases: 88M (21M); Deaths: 1.8M (365K); CFR: 2.0%

Post #93: Slow Vaccine Rollout

Jan. 8, 2021

As a former 11-year CDC federal employee, I can attest that bureaucracy is slow. The government does not move at the speed of business when it comes to logistics & innovation. Case and point: vaccine distribution. We were promised 20 million vaccinations by the end of 2020. To date, there have been 6.5 million given, only 29% of the 21 million doses distributed. California gave the most shots (2.9M). North Dakota used the most of their allotment (62%). States' lack of cold storage capacity, training, planning of distribution logistics, and any number of local snafus has slowed the rollout. The feds have admitted failure & pledged to do better. Their controversial strategy to hold back vaccines is being revisited. Ultimately, to boost gains from public health precautions and personal responsibility, vaccines must move from ultra-cold storage into the arms of Americans. Despite a deluge of band-aid warriors posting selfies all over social media, there has been persistent vaccine hesitancy even among health professionals. COVID vaccines have always been a moonshot, but success has been crippled by the lack of a coordinated national response. Time will tell if this changes with the Biden team.

Cases: 88M (21M); Deaths: 1.9M (365K); CFR: 2.2%

Post #94: Complicit

Jan. 10, 2020

What does the violent siege on our nation's Capital have to do with (mis)managing the raging pandemic? Obviously, toppling the seat of democracy would cripple lawmaker's ability to pass additional COVID relief & funding urgently needed to bolster states' capacity for testing and vaccinations. But also, two parallel acts of complicity reinforce disastrous, if not avoidable, outcomes. Both were fueled by a rhetoric of denial and falsehoods. Both were led by an outgoing president determined to downplay the threat of COVID amid peaking numbers. By protesting face masks, endorsing unorthodox therapies, cheering those refusing stay at home orders, retweeting inflammatory gibberish, dog-whistling to white nationalists, Trump's self-serving actions have simultaneously managed to force the nation to take its eyes off record-setting death tolls and shift focus to his desperate efforts to stay in office. His instigation of the latest superspreading insurrection led to 5 deaths, dozens of arrests, and will undoubtedly result in thousands of more infections. It would be refreshing to have leaders from both parties eager to double down on thwarting COVID rather than to advance their own political fortunes. This is exhausting.

Cases: 89M (22M); Deaths: 1.9M (372K); CFR: 2.1%

Post #95: There's an App for That

Feb. 8, 2021

Why do our most vulnerable struggle to find COVID-19 resources? They go online & call and get confusing information, a busy signal, or the run-around. Some secure a slot but are turned away when they arrive. Why so complicated? I recently traveled to the middle east. I had to show proof of a negative PCR test prior to boarding my flight & was required to download a national testing app upon arrival. The app informed my quarantine period and listed the nearest drive-thru location for a FREE test. On the day of my appointment, I grabbed a taxi, drove through the winding lanes of a large parking lot, and rolled down my window at the testing booth. Someone from the health dept. scanned my QR code then swabbed my throat. The process took all of 15 minutes. The app immediately updated my status, and my negative test result was posted 2-days later. How easy was that? There's a similar process for receiving vaccinations, although not offered by drive-thru, yet. Why can't we do that? Granted, Healthcare.gov (the Obamacare website) was a debacle. But should states have to struggle with logistics when there's an app for that? To navigate the pandemic, America must work smarter. It's embarrassing.

Cases: 106M (27M); Deaths: 2.3M (463K); CFR: 2.2%

Post #96: Double Mask, Doubly Good?

Feb. 9, 2021

Here we go again with the masks. Remember when this all began? We were told to leave the masks for the health professionals. Well, at least the medical-grade N-95 versions. Then we were instructed to use home-rigged cloth coverings. We later learned about which masks work, and those that can make matters worse (no valves, people). It was initially touted that masks protected others, not yourself. That is before the authorities arrived at the logical conclusion that they did both. Today, it's generally accepted that masks reduce air-sprayed transmissions by up to 50 percent. That's great. Only now I'm hearing that we may want to double mask. Excuse me? I'm a strong proponent of masks. I follow the science. But double masking? Why not triple mask, Dr. Fauci? Let's not get carried away here. This recommendation no doubt stems more from desperation than science. We have not seen the vaccination penetration we need for herd immunity. Folks are fatigued at the slow progress. However, I believe that a single, well-fitted, mask consistently worn will do the trick. Combined with social distancing, hand hygiene, and vaccinations (for those so inclined), we will get to the other side.

Cases: 106M (27M); Deaths: 2.3M (463K); CFR: 2.2%

Post #97: Reporting Side Effects

Feb. 13, 2021

Potential side effects are a common reason for vaccine hesitancy. Some fear the vaccine will cause COVID. It won't. Others worry about long-term complications. Life-threatening allergic reactions are rare but can happen, usually within minutes of the shot. More often, vaccinated people report fatigue, fever, chills, headache, muscle, and joint pains, often within 2-7 days. These symptoms result from your body's immune response to the vaccine. Vaccine makers & healthcare providers are required by law to report serious side effects to the CDC. But you can too! Here are two ways to report your experience. First, register for V-safe. It's not an app, but rather a smartphone-based tool that uses text messaging to provide health check-ins after you receive a vaccination. Bonus: it also reminds you when to get your second dose! Serious complaints to V-safe will prompt a direct call from CDC. Unfortunately, so far less than 10% of those receiving the vaccine have registered. Second, if you suspect a bad experience related to the vaccine you can report it using CDC's online reporting system called VAERS. There's also a writeable PDF form. Either way, you choose to report it, report it.

Cases: 108M (27M); Deaths: 2.3M (484K); CFR: 2.1%

Post #98: Coming to Your Local Pharmacy

Feb. 15, 2021

It seems like there's a CVS on every corner, right? That's because there practically is. For example, more than 70% of Americans live within 3-miles of a CVS pharmacy. There are nearly 10,000 CVS stores and almost the same number of Walgreens stores. Between CVS, Walgreens, Walmart & Rite Aid, even the most vulnerable communities—those at highest risk—have physical access. This is critically important because these retail pharmacies have recently been enlisted as partners in the federal program to provide COVID vaccines. Although they will only be given one million doses, to begin with, this makes good sense because many of these stores have been providing COVID testing. Their convenient locations and store hours may help put an end to the runaround when it comes to finding a location. The 1 million doses will be spread over a few dozen states, but the program is expected to expand depending on vaccine supply. You'll likely need an appointment, and you still have to wait your turn in line, but it's refreshing to see the government leveraging existing infrastructure as points of distribution. This will not only increase access but will decompress hospitals and clinics. Smart.

Cases: 109M (27M); Deaths: 2.4M (485K); CFR: 2.2%

Post #99: Vaccines Safe, So Far

Feb. 18, 2021

The debate about vaccine safety is ongoing, but the statistics are telling. So far, there have been about 1,200 deaths among people who were vaccinated. Fortunately, none of these deaths have been linked to the vaccine. People die. Actually, roughly 7,800 deaths every day in the U.S., most often from heart disease and cancer. These diseases increase with age. Seniors over 65 years & in nursing homes are among the first to be vaccinated. So, this checks out. Life-threatening allergic reactions can happen, but are rare, occurring in 5 people for every million receiving the vaccine. However, this is a known risk with any vaccine. They usually happen within minutes which is why you are required to be monitored immediately after your shot. According to a recent study, most were treated in the Emergency Dept., few required hospitalization. Reported allergies included bee stings, wasp stings, eggs, shellfish, nuts, antibiotics, and other medications. Bottom line: as long as you disclose your allergy history, the short-term risks from vaccination appear to be minuscule. Given that vaccines may represent the off-ramp to this nightmare, the benefits would appear to outweigh the risks.

Cases: 110M (27M); Deaths: 2.4M (490K); CFR: 2.2%

Post #100: 500,000

Feb. 23, 2021

One year ago, I posted the first blog in this series. At the time there were 60 cases and zero deaths. We've just reached a half-million. For perspective, consider this: if every death came from the city of Miami, its entire population would be wiped out. By contrast, seasonal flu causes up to 60,000 deaths per year & the H1N1 pandemic of 2009, just under 13,000. The worse pandemic on record (flu pandemic of 1918) killed 675,000 Americans. Sadly, we're on pace to surpass that number. Experts project we'll hit 600,000 deaths by mid-June. We hope that the death curve will flatten with widespread uptake of the vaccines, but COVID fatigue & vaccine hesitancy might dictate otherwise. The needed 75% immunity for herd protection is a moonshot. Optimistically, immunity from vaccines & natural infection may be approaching 30%. And with the already spotty vaccine distribution disrupted by extreme weather, the Biden team faces uphill sledding (no pun intended). Sometimes progress is slower than we want. But maybe the devastation of COVID will be more than a wake-up call. Perhaps it will be a rallying call. There's no better time for Americans to end the uncivil war and collectively take care of one another.

Cases: 111M (28M); Deaths: 2.4M (500K); CFR: 2.2%

Total COVID-19 deaths in the U.S. through February 2021

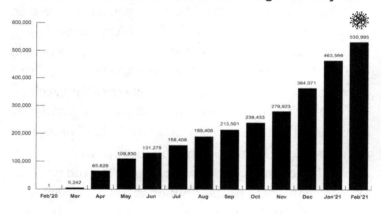

Source: Worldometer

AFTERWORD

In the months to follow, the pandemic seemed to mirror a race with two competitors. The first was the coronavirus that was clearly winning. In fact, it was so far out front that at times it appeared that it would never be caught. The virus clearly had a head start. It had crept into the US undetected, then by cruise ship. And despite its arrival, our national leaders denied out loud any possible threat. We would later learn that behind the scenes, Trump and company knew better, but simply chose to ignore the long-standing playbook. Instead, the administration opted for the bury-our-head-in-the-sand, and all will be well by Easter, response. As a result, the case counts continued to march ahead at a blistering pace. From the record-setting high of 28 million cases of COVID-19 in February, the US case count rose by about 2 million every month: March ended with 30 million, April ended with 32 million, and May with 34 million. As the virus continued to circulate in the US and around the world, more than a dozen new variants emerged. While some of these variants were of interest, many were of high consequence as they were presumed to be more contagious and likely more lethal.

By mid-June, we eclipsed 600,000 COVID deaths in the US according to the CDC and other official trackers. This was the highest national death toll from a pandemic since the Spanish flu of 1918 which killed roughly 675,000 people. However, just a month prior, scientists estimated the actual death count was closer to 900,000. Their models suggested that official counts underestimated deaths by as much as 57%. By examining excess deaths (i.e., deaths greater than what would have been predicted during a nonpandemic year), researchers were able to attribute most of these to COVID, factoring in extra deaths caused by increased opioid overdoses or those resulting from deferred health care (e.g., people who died because they did not or could not get their health needs met because healthcare workers were too overwhelmed by COVID cases). If this model holds, instead of 600,000 deaths through mid-June it would be closer to 942,000, far exceeding those from the scourge in 1918.

Meanwhile, vaccine development, the other competitor in this race, was stumbling out of the starting blocks trying desperately to catch up. In fairness, the vaccine was developed at relative warp speed. By utilizing technology available decades earlier, government subsidies, and international collaboration, three vaccines (Pfizer, Moderna, and Johnson and Johnson) were widely available to all groups by the spring. Unanticipated hurdles related to vaccine distribution logistics, traditional vaccine hesitancy by some communities, and conspiracy theories hampered the campaign. Like ethnic and racial minority communities, rural residents and Republicans were less likely to get vaccinated although for completely different reasons. At the time of writing, 23% of Blacks and 28% of Latinos are fully vaccinated compared to 32% of whites. However, whereas white people received a higher share of vaccinations compared to their share of COVID cases, the opposite was true for Blacks and Latinos across most states. Fortunately, vaccine hesitancy appears to be waning among vulnerable groups (and all Americans) over time.

We are not out of the woods by any means. The virus is still reeling out of control in other regions of the world, including parts of Asia, Southern Africa, and South America. A threat anywhere is a threat everywhere. But we're finally seeing light at the end of the tunnel. Nearly half of the nation is fully vaccinated at the time of writing, and almost 80% of seniors aged 65 years and older. Now that COVID vaccines are approved for teens and will soon be approved for children aged 5 and older, I would expect vaccination rates to continue to rise. That said, it is unlikely that we will ever achieve herd immunity which would require an overall population vaccination rate of at least 70%. However, 34 million people were infected naturally with the virus. Presumably, we can add another 10% to the nation's herd immunity because these people received immunity (at least for a period of time) resulting from their infection.

In the final analysis, it will take time to reconcile all the numbers, rates, and ratios. It may take longer still to fully grasp the genetic pressures or circumstances that led to the emergence of this cunning novel coronavirus. What we cannot be confused about, nor underestimate, is the importance of competent leadership at all levels of government, the importance of trusting the science (even as it evolves), cross-jurisdictional collaboration, and personal and collective responsibility. Following the loss of no fewer than 600,000 lives, with millions of survivors left with significant medical complications (i.e., long-haulers), and incalculable psychological and economic trauma, the stakes have proved to be high. There has always been a playbook for outbreaks, epidemics, and pandemics. Thanks to COVID-19, we have added valuable pages to the script. To not follow the playbook and heed the lessons learned is to risk repeating mistakes during the next pandemic which will surely come, and sooner rather than later.

GLOSSARY OF TERMS

Active immunity. occurs when our immune system responsible for protecting us is exposed to a pathogen: *the duration of active immunity following COVID is uncertain.*

Airborne diseases. are bacteria or viruses that are most commonly transmitted through small respiratory droplets: *coronavirus is an airborne disease that can spread by droplets when someone sneezes, coughs, laughs, or otherwise exhales in some way.*

Antibodies. also called immunoglobulin. a protective protein produced by the immune system in response to the presence of a foreign substance, called an antigen: *coronavirus antibodies develop several weeks after infection.*

Antibody test. detects the antibody produced by the body in response to the virus: *a positive antibody test for COVID means a person was infected by a coronavirus in the past.*

Antigen. a toxin or other foreign substance which induces an immune response in the body, including the production of antibodies: *the COVID virus is an antigen.*

Antigen test. detects proteins that are part of the coronavirus: *an antigen test measures coronavirus proteins in the blood or saliva sample.*

Aerosol. a suspension of liquid and/or solid particles: *coronavirus particles can be found in fine aerosol and inhaled by close contacts.*

Attack rate. the percentage of an at-risk population that contracts the disease during a specified time interval: *the attack rate for coronavirus is probably higher among the elderly.*

Attenuated. having been reduced in force or value; in case of vaccine, reduced or weaken virulence: *most vaccines are made from either inactivated (dead) or attenuated virus.*

Attenuated vaccine. also called live attenuated vaccine (LAV). is a vaccine developed by reducing the virulence of the pathogen: *vaccines for measles, mumps, rubella are live attenuated vaccines.*

Case fatality rate. also called case fatality ratio or case fatality risk. is the proportion of deaths from a certain disease compared to the total number of people diagnosed with the disease for a particular period: *the case fatality rate for COVID is around two percent.*

Cluster. refers to an aggregation of cases grouped in place and time that are suspected to be greater than the number expected: *early on, there were a number of COVID clusters in Washington state associated with nursing homes.*

Communicable disease. one that is spread from one person to another through a variety of ways that include contact with blood and bodily fluids, breathing in an airborne virus: *most respiratory viruses are communicable diseases.*

Contact tracing. the process of identifying all people that a COVID-19 patient has come in contact with in the last two weeks: *contact tracing is critical to controlling the spread of COVID.*

Convalescent plasma. the therapy uses blood (rich with protective antibodies) from people who've recovered from an illness to help others recover: *there was mild success with treating COVID with convalescent plasma before the availability of a vaccine.*

Coronavirus. abbreviated CoV. is a large family of viruses that cause illnesses ranging from the common cold to more severe diseases: *both Middle East Respiratory Syndrome (MERS-CoV) and Severe Acute Respiratory Syndrome (SARS-CoV) are examples of coronaviruses.*

COVID. shorthand for COronaVIrus Disease. the clinical illness that results from being infected by a coronavirus: *infection with the novel coronavirus may cause asymptomatic COVID-19.*

COVID-19. the clinical disease that results from infection with the 2019 novel coronavirus (SARS-CoV-2): *common symptoms of COVID-19 include fever, cough, shortness of breath.*

Cross protection. implies clinically significant protection against infection/disease due to an immune response elicited against a related organism: *we think the COVID-19 vaccines confer cross-protection for new emergent variants of the virus.*

Emergency Use Authorization. abbreviated EUA. a mechanism to fast-track the availability of medical countermeasures like vaccines, during public health emergencies: *COVID vaccines have been given EUA by the FDA because they are deemed safe and are urgently needed.*

Epidemic. a widespread occurrence of an infectious disease in a community at a particular time: *COVID began as an epidemic in Wuhan, China.*

Epidemic curve. also called epi curve or epidemiological curve is a statistical chart used in epidemiology to visualize the onset of a disease outbreak: *the epi-curve in the US has flattened following widespread vaccinations.*

Epidemiology. the study of how often diseases (infectious and non-infectious) occur in different groups of people and why: *epidemiology is a common concentration in graduate schools of public health.*

Herd immunity. occurs when a large portion of a community (the herd) becomes immune to a disease, making the spread of disease from person to person unlikely: *the US may never reach herd immunity for COVID.*

Hotspot. areas of elevated incidence or prevalence, higher transmission efficiency or risk, or higher probability of disease emergence: *hotspots and clusters are often used interchangeably.*

Immunity. the body's defense system to fight against antigens and protect the body: *immunity to certain infections can wane with age requiring a booster shot.*

Immunology. the study of the immune system: *I spent the summer of 1991 at the CDC studying immunology.*

Incubation period. the number of days between when you're infected with something and when you might see symptoms: *the incubation period for COVID is 14 days.*

Innate immunity. natural immunity. is the nonspecific defense mechanisms that we're born with to keep harmful substances from entering the body, including barriers such as skin and mucous membranes: *SARS-CoV-2 easily evades our innate immunity.*

Isolation. separates sick people with a contagious disease from people who are not sick: *isolation is an important mitigation strategy to slow the spread of COVID.*

Mitigation strategies. steps are taken to reduce the risk, the severity of the impact, and/or probability of the occurrence: *mitigation strategies for COVID include hand washing, physical distancing, and wearing facemasks.*

mRNA vaccine. a new type of vaccine to protect against infectious diseases by teaching our cells how to make a protein (or piece of a protein) that triggers an immune response inside our bodies: *both Pfizer and Moderna vaccines are mRNA vaccines.*

Mutation. a change in a DNA sequence often due to errors occurring during the virus's copying process: *mutations are what have led to new variants of coronavirus.*

Outbreak. a sudden rise in the incidence of a disease, usually compared to the baseline rate: *most measles outbreaks are related to communities that do not vaccinate their children.*

Pandemic. an epidemic that has spread over several countries or continents, usually affecting a large number of people: *a global epidemic is a pandemic.*

Passive immunity. occurs when we are protected from a pathogen by immunity gained from someone else: *one way to get passive immunity is by receiving convalescent plasma from a person that survived COVID.*

Pathogen. a microorganism that causes, or can cause, disease: *common pathogens include viruses and bacteria.*

PCR test. a polymerase chain reaction (PCR) test is performed to detect genetic material (RNA) from a specific organism: *the PCR test result confirmed he was infected with coronavirus at the time of the test.*

Quarantine. separates and restricts the movement of people who were exposed to a contagious disease to see if they become sick: *quarantine is a common mitigation strategy, especially for life-threatening, contagious, diseases.*

RNA test. see also PCR test. a test to detect RNA genetic material: *the RNA test can be positive before COVID antibodies forming.*

Rona. urban slang for coronavirus: *she avoided the house party because of fear of getting the Rona.*

SARS-CoV-2. Sudden Acute Respiratory Syndrome-Coronavirus-2, the virus that causes COVID: *the official name for novel coronavirus is SARS-CoV-2.*

Social distancing. to maintain a safe or appropriate distance from other people, especially to slow the spread of a contagious illness or disease: *out of an abundance of caution, we're socially distancing ourselves from friends and extended family.*

Vaccine. A vaccine can confer active immunity against a specific harmful agent by stimulating the immune system to attack the agent: *more than half of US adults have received the COVID vaccine.*

Vaccine effectiveness. Effectiveness refers to how well a vaccine performs in the real world: *although the Pfizer vaccine had a 95% efficacy in the study, the effectiveness was closer to 80%.*

Vaccine efficacy. the degree to which a vaccine prevents disease (and possibly also transmission) under study conditions, comparing a vaccinated group with a placebo group: *the FDA set a 50% vaccine efficacy threshold for emergency use authorization of COVID vaccines.*

Vaccinology. the science of vaccines, and historically includes basic science, immunogens, the host immune response, delivery strategies and technologies, manufacturing, and clinical evaluation.

Variant. a form of something that differs in some respect from other forms of the same thing: *there are now several coronavirus variants in circulation that may be more deadly than the original.*

Vaccine mutation. random genetic copying errors in a virus that changes the virus, leading to alterations in the virus' surface proteins or antigens: *viral mutations led to variant types of coronavirus that may be more deadly.*

Viral shedding. when infected individuals shed viral particles while they talk, exhale, eat, and perform other normal daily activities: *people with mild COVID infection stop shedding virus 10 days after symptoms begin.*

BIBLIOGRAPHY

Ahmad, F. B., & Anderson, R. N. (2021, May 11). *The Leading Causes of Death in the US for 2020.* JAMA. https://jamanetwork.com/journals/jama/fullarticle/2778234.

AJMC Staff. (2021, January 2). *A Timeline of COVID-19 Developments in 2020.* https://www.ajmc.com/view/a-timeline-of-covid19-developments-in-2020.

Bikales, J. (2020, November 21). *How risky was that Napa Valley party Gavin Newsom attended?* San Francisco Chronicle. https://www.sfchronicle.com/health/article/How-risky-was-that-Napa-party-Gavin-Newsom-15744050.php.

Cable News Network. (2020, March 17). *Right Now with Brianna Keilar. Coronavirus response.* CNN. http://transcripts.cnn.com/TRANSCRIPTS/2003/17/crn.02.html.

Cable News Network. (2020, June 9). *This Hour with Kate Bolduan. Upsurge in COVID-19 Cases.* CNN. http://www.cnn.com/TRANSCRIPTS/2006/08/cnr.06.html

Centers for Disease Control and Prevention. (n.d.). *CDC COVID Data Tracker.* https://covid.cdc.gov/covid-data-tracker/#datatracker-home.

Centers for Disease Control and Prevention. (n.d.). *Coronavirus Disease 2019 (COVID-19).* https://www.cdc.gov/coronavirus/2019-ncov/index.html.

Entis, L. (2020, September 4). *Three steps organizations can take to address health disparities - Features.* MM+M - Medical Marketing and Media. https://www.mmm-online.com/home/channel/features/three-steps-organizations-can-take-to-address-health-disparities/.

Goldman, L. (2020, March 15). *What are the rules of social distancing?* Vox. https://www.vox.com/2020/3/15/21179296/coronavirus-covid-19-social-distancing-bored-pandemic-quarantine-ethics.

Hasbrouck, L. (2020, April 24). *Returning to business after COVID-19.* The Hill. https://thehill.com/opinion/finance/494525-returning-to-business-after-covid-19.

Hasbrouck, L. (2020, May 7). *Commentary: Gov. Pritzker has the right idea, but a vaccine will not save us.* Chicago Tribune. https://www.chicagotribune.com/opinion/commentary/ct-opinion-coronavirus-vaccine-illinois-20200507-bfkagw7dyfehhn3wsptt3rdh7i-story.html.

Hasbrouck, L. (2020, December 9). *Top 10 things Black Americans need to know about the vaccine.* TheGrio. https://thegrio.com/2020/12/09/10-things-black-americans-need-to-know-vaccine/.

Hasbrouck, L. (2021, February 17). *10 more things Black Americans should know about the COVID-19 vaccine.* TheGrio. https://thegrio.com/2021/02/17/10-things-black-americans-should-know-about-vaccine/.

Kovensky, J. (2020, June 10). *These Factors Will Determine What the Next COVID Outbreak Will Look Like.* Talking Points Memo. https://talkingpointsmemo.com/muckraker/these-factors-will-determine-what-the-next-covid-outbreak-will-look-like.

Kovensky, J. (2020, September 14). *'Disastrous': Why It's So Damaging for Trump Admin to Doctor The CDC's COVID Reports.* Talking Points Memo. https://talkingpointsmemo.com/muckraker/disastrous-why-its-so-damaging-for-trump-admin-to-doctor-the-cdcs-covid-reports.

Mahr, J., & Dardick, H. (2020, March 27). *Illinois' pandemic plan anticipated shortages and surges, anxiety and death. Now the public is seeing how the state meets the test.* Chicago Tribune. https://www.chicagotribune.com/coronavirus/ct-illinois-pandemic-plan-coronavirus-20200327-367axxfjjjfb3jgtkfdpoauj4m-story.html.

Mallenbaum, C. (2020, June 11). *Should you wear a face mask to the gym? A look at the debate.* USA Today. https://www.usatoday.com/story/life/2020/06/10/face-mask-gym-debate-coronavirus-safety-precaution/3161272001/.

Mallenbaum, C. (2020, March 13). *SoulCycle reduces class sizes by 50% amid coronavirus; Here's how to stay healthy at gyms.* USA Today. https://www.usatoday.com/story/life/health-wellness/2020/03/03/coronavirus-guide-proper-gym-etiquette-during-outbreak/4946980002/.

Montague, C. Y. A. (2021, March 21). *Journalists need to go beyond Tuskegee when reporting on vaccines among Black Americans.* Center for Health Journalism. https://centerforhealthjournalism.org/2021/03/11/journalists-need-go-beyond-tuskegee-when-reporting-vaccines-among-black-americans.

Muccari, R., Chow, D., & Murphy, J. (2021, January 1). *Coronavirus timeline: Tracking the critical moments of Covid-19.* NBCNews.com. https://www.nbcnews.com/health/health-news/coronavirus-timeline-tracking-critical-moments-covid-19-n1154341.

New York Times Staff. (2020, January 28). *Coronavirus World Map: Tracking the Global Outbreak.* The New York Times. https://www.nytimes.com/interactive/2021/world/covid-cases.html.

O'Donnell, J. (2020, April 29). *Tackling poverty in a coronavirus-induced economic downturn: Is it too risky or the right thing to do?* USA Today. https://www.usatoday.com/story/news/ health/2020/04/28/coronavirus-poverty-fight-public-health/5164303002/.

O'Donnell, J. (2020, March 3). *'This is not sustainable': Public health departments, decimated by funding cuts, scramble against coronavirus.* USA Today. https:// www.usatoday.com/story/news/health/2020/03/02/ coronavirus-response-depleted-public-health-departments-scramble-respond/4868693002/.

Riga, K. (2020, October 26). *Pence Hijacks 'Essential Worker' Title To Excuse Himself From Quarantining.* Talking Points Memo. https://talkingpointsmemo. com/news/pence-covid-essential-worker-short-election.

Sullivan, B. (2021, May 6). *New Study Estimates More Than 900,000 People Have Died of COVID-19 In U.S.* NPR. https://www.npr.org/sections/ coronavirus-live-updates/2021/05/06/994287048/ new-study-estimates-more-than-900-000-people-have-died-of-covid-19-in-u-s.

U.S. Food and Drug Administration. (n.d.). *Emergency Use Authorization for Vaccines Explained.* U.S. Food and Drug Administration. https://www.fda.gov/ vaccines-blood-biologics/vaccines/emergency-use-authorization-vaccines-explained.

University of Minnesota School of Public Health. (2020, December 3). *Episode 4: Race & Public*

Health: Tuskegee to COVID-19 – If not now, when? Racism: A 400-year public health emergency. School of Public Health. https://www.sph.umn.edu/podcast/series-2/episode-4-race-and-public-health-tuskegee-covid-19/.

Vuocolo, A. (2021, March 29). *Going Out This Memorial Day? Best Practices for a Safe Holiday.* Cheddar. https://cheddar.com/media/going-out-this-memorial-day-best-practices-for-a-safe-holiday.

Worldometer. (n.d.). United States COVID Cases. Worldometer. https://www.worldometers.info/coronavirus/country/us/.

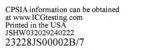

9 781956 780352